The Teeth in Health and Disease

THE TEETH

THE TEETH

IN

HEALTH AND DISEASE

BY

GEORGE READ MATLAND

AND

THOMAS COLLIER MATLAND

DENTAL SURGEONS

ILLUSTRATED

LONDON

WARD, LOCK AND CO., LIMITED

NEW YORK AND MELBOURNE

1904

Preface

IN presenting this book to their patients the authors trust that it may be the means of spreading some useful knowledge of the dental organs and lead to a due appreciation of the important function the teeth perform in the maintenance of health. A deplorable lack of information upon this subject is displayed even by people who are otherwise well informed and who possess considerable general intelligence. Beyond the purely advertising pamphlet, the popular literature on the teeth is extremely limited, and it is hoped by the authors that the following pages will help to remedy the deficiency in this respect. They have endeavoured to give in as concise a manner as possible sufficient information to enable their readers to take reasonable care of their teeth and to recognize when it is desirable to consult a dental practitioner. In order to do this considerable prominence has been given to diseases of the teeth and gums and especially those arising from dental neglect, and from the presence of diseased and putrid roots in the mouth.

Concerning the use of anesthetics in dentistry the authors have endeavoured to afford infor-mation which will prove of general interest, and regarding cocaine anesthesia they can fairly claim to speak with authority, as their experience in the use of this agent is very extensive.

The chapter on hygiene of the mouth con-tains much information on the preservation of the teeth and on the course to be followed to render the mouth clean and healthy, to which are added some remarks on dentifrices, etc.

The concluding portion of the work re-ferring to artificial teeth should prove of service to those who are forced to adopt these useful appliances.

1, 3, AND 5, FINSBURY PAVEMENT,
LONDON, E.C.
May 1st, 1902.

Contents

Introductory

IT is impossible to overrate the value of a good set of teeth even if their use in the mastication of the food is alone considered, but when in addition we estimate their services in assisting vocalization, and the necessity of their preservation in order to maintain the natural contour of the face, it is an obvious duty on the part of all to do their utmost to avoid those causes that lead to the premature destruction and decay of these useful organs. The preservation of the health of the mouth and teeth is essential to the general well-being. Disease of the body involves an unhealthy condition of the mouth, and is manifested by perceptible changes in the tongue, gum, lips, and mucous membrane.

A diseased and unwholesome condition of the mouth cannot fail to act prejudicially on the bodily welfare. The pain and consequent loss of rest arising from decayed teeth are often very exhausting, and reduce seriously the vital energies. The loss of the power of mastication directly affects the digestion, which is further impaired by the vitiation of the secretions of the mouth brought about by a congested and inflamed state of the gums. The constant swallowing of the purulent discharge produced by broken-down roots and decayed and abscessed teeth tends to irritate the stomach, while the air inhaled into the lungs is made offensive and is loaded with septic impurities which prevent it exercising its best influence on the delicate air cells of which these organs are built up, and on the blood which depends for its quality on the purity of the air respired.

It is probable there has now been for several generations a progressive deterioration in the human dental outfit among civilized races.

Structurally defective and decayed teeth and ill-developed jaws and irregular teeth are more prevalent, and the absorption of the sockets, recession of the gums, and consequent falling out of the teeth, more frequently met with long before the attainment of the period of middle age, instead of being practically unknown until an advanced age is reached.

If this dental degeneration is to be successfully combated, it must be not alone nor chiefly through the manipulative skill of dental operators, but by a more thorough appreciation by the people of its causes and of the means by which they may be avoided.

Matters of much less importance to personal

appearance, of vastly less account to individual comfort, and of far smaller moment to health and life, are made the subjects of constant study and care, while the teeth are utterly neglected until disease and decay have so far progressed that their extraction is the only possible treatment.

Patients defer consulting a dentist until their mouth is in an almost hopelessly diseased state, their gums inflamed and irritated by a number of ulcerated roots, and possessing only decayed teeth with large cavities in which decomposing food remains for weeks and months, rendering the breath unbearably offensive. Neuralgic pains, abscesses, diseased jaws, with disfiguring wounds on the face and neck, dyspeptic troubles, tumours, and abnormal growths of various kinds, and protracted diseases of the nose, ears, throat, and eyes, are often the result of a neglected mouth and diseased teeth, although the true cause of such diseases may be frequently overlooked both by the patient and his medical adviser.

It is absolutely true, as a writer in *The British Journal of Dental Science* of October 15th, 1901, remarks that :—

" Hundreds and thousands of people are going about with decayed teeth, carrying with them so many small cesspools in their mouths,

filled with fetid abominations of putrid food
debris, with its teeming population of micro-
organisms, daily swallowing these putrefac-
tions, and absorbing the pus. Many cases
of septic diseases are due to dental caries.
Its effects may be manifested in multifarious
ways. Many of the so-called ' scrofulous '
scars of the neck have had their starting point
in carious teeth. The usual complaint by
patients that fresh air will give them face ache
is in most cases due to uncared-for carious
teeth. Many laryngeal and pharyngeal (throat)
troubles have their origin in the same cause.
A man with a decayed molar hardly ever has a
clean tongue."

˙ The *Journal* of the British Dental Association, commenting upon the annual conference
of the " Health Society," remarks :—

" The subject of ' health ' can hardly be
adequately discussed without a certain amount
of attention to the dental aspect of the
question.

" We believe half of London to be rendered
unhealthy for the want of systematic instruction in dental sanitation. Hundreds of thousands of people go about night and day
creating insanitary conditions by means of
emanations from decaying stumps, chronic
abscesses, inflamed gums eaten into by tartar,

and last—not least—the noxious gases formed in the stomachs of those unfortunates who, destitute of proper masticatory apparatus, cannot digest their food.

"The poor and dirty dwellers in the slums have much to learn concerning health and sanitation, and no doubt simple and long-established axioms will require much demonstrating and explaining before they are brought home to the dregs of the population, and the general ignorance about the teeth would form a capital subject for an energetic and enthusiastic philanthropist.

"We all know what the results of tartar are, yet we would venture to say that tartar exists to a very detrimental extent in the purlieus of London in the mouths of the uncleanly poor, and thereby not only they themselves are injured in health, but the very air is rendered less fit for respiration and a more efficient medium for the spread of disease.

"The effect may be seen in the greeny-white faces, the dwarfed stature, sunken chests, sore eyes, and rickety limbs, that people these districts. The boon of model dwellinghouses might with advantage be combined with the introduction of tooth brushes, and instruction how to use them.

"If the lowest strata of society could be

restored to the blessings of cleanliness and a good digestion, many grievances would disappear of themselves, and the life of London would be healthier and happier.

"We would urge, then, upon the consideration of the Health Society that their scheme is imperfect if the mouth—the greatest factor in the relative impurity or purity of the body—is allowed to remain in an unwholesome condition."

The
Mastication and Insalivation of Food.

GOOD health demands thorough digestion: thorough digestion demands thorough mastication, and thorough mastication demands sound and healthy teeth. Ulcerated roots and decayed teeth, an inflamed mouth and vitiated saliva, are poorly fitted to supply the stomach with food that can be properly digested and assimilated. An eminent writer, speaking upon this subject, says :—

"The stomach may be compared to a stove: the food to the fuel consumed by the stove, and life to the heat given off by the glowing coals. The stomach is an excellent stove and will burn much bad fuel; but have a care lest it rebel and the fire be extinguished."

To maintain a vigorous and sustained vital

glow, a suitable aliment must be supplied and it must be thoroughly ground by the teeth and moistened by the fluid called the saliva, which is the first of the digestive fluids that the food meets in its progress through the body. The introduction of food into the mouth results in the discharge from a number of glands of an increased quantity of saliva which, mixing with the food, assists the teeth in reducing it to a fit condition for the digestive organs to continue the work of breaking it up, separating and assimilating its nutritive constituents.

The saliva is secreted by three pairs of glands placed symmetrically on the right and left sides of the mouth; these are the parotid glands which are situated immediately below and in front of the ear, the sub-maxillary glands, which are placed under the angle of the lower jaw, and the sub-lingual glands which are found under the tongue in the fleshy part of the mouth. All of these glands communicate with the mouth by special conduits or ducts, those of the parotid, known as Steno's ducts, opening inside the mouth, immediately opposite the second molar teeth, while the sub-maxillary and the sub-lingual have their outlets in the floor of the mouth beneath the tongue. The secretions of the various glands differ: that of the parotid is most abundant and is a clear and limpid fluid. Its principal function is to moisten the food and reduce it to the required consistency. The thick ropy fluid secreted by the sub-maxillary gland promotes the solution of the soluble substances and specially impresses the nerves of taste, while that of the sub-lingual gland lubricates the food and facilitates its passage down the pharynx. The parotid glands are the chief source of the moisture that flows into the mouth during continuous speaking; and when inflamed they constitute the disease known as mumps.

The numerous mucous glands which exist in the floor and roof of the mouth, tongue, gums, and cheeks also add their quota to the moisture of the mouth; they secrete a somewhat turbid slightly viscid fluid having a faint acid reaction (mucus).

The mixture of all these secretions constitute the saliva, which is a thick, glairy, generally frothy and slightly turbid fluid consisting of about 99 per cent of water. Its reaction in health is alkaline, especially when the secretion is abundant. Saliva contains but few solids; of these about half consist of salts and half of ptyalin and other organic principles. Ptyalin is the active principle of the saliva, which plays an important part in digestion;

it has the power of converting starch into grape sugar, which is the first step in a series of chemical processes (digestion) by which the food is prepared for the uses of the economy. That the action of the saliva upon starchy foods is of great importance becomes ap-

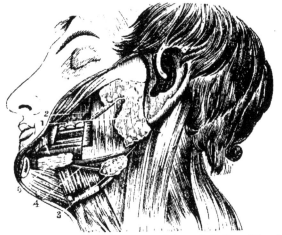

Fig. 1.—Dissection showing position of Saliva Glands.
1. Parotid (near the ear).
2. Duct of Steno (leading from parotid gland to mouth).
3. Sub-maxillary gland (beneath the jaw).
4. Duct of sub-maxillary gland.
5. Sub-lingual (beneath the tongue).

parent when it is understood that starch as such is insoluble and would therefore be not only valueless as nutriment but a positive burden to the digestive organs, while the sugar into which it is converted by the saliva is readily soluble and nutritious. The

quantity of saliva discharged into the mouth
varies with the condition of the food introduced,
being abundant in proportion to the dryness
of the food.   Its secretion varies also with
the varying health of the body.   It is much
diminished and sometimes almost suspended
by fear, anxiety, or other depressing emotions.
In diseased conditions of the general system
its character is variously modified, becoming
acid or excessively alkaline ; acting upon the
soft tissues of the mouth, causing soreness and
ulceration, and upon the teeth, causing their
disintegration.   Thus it often happens that
during a severe illness very serious inroads
are made upon the integrity of the structures
of the teeth which are attributed frequently
and erroneously to the medicine taken.

The acts of mastication and deglutition are
more complex than they at first sight appear.
The food, first divided into pieces of suitable
size by the front teeth, is passed back to the
molars, which by their grinding action rapidly
convert it into a pulpy mass.   The tongue
and cheeks participate by passing the food
backward and forward over the grinding surfaces of the teeth, and preventing any portion of
it escaping titeration.   Having been sufficiently
masticated the food is rolled into a rough bolus
or ball by the tongue, lubricated by the saliva,

and is passed backward towards the gullet or esophagus. The processes up to this point

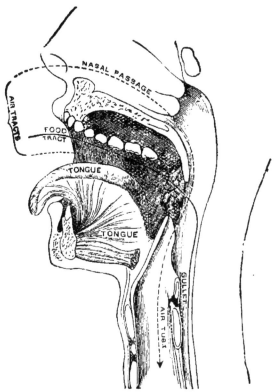

FIG. 2.—Diagram of Food and Air Tracts.
The solid line through mouth and gullet represents the course taken by food and drink; the dotted lines through mouth, nasal passages, and air-tube represent the course taken by the air.

have been voluntary, dependent on the will, but as the food reaches the gullet an involuntary muscular action is excited and the food is seized and passed downwards into the stomach by muscles which act independently of the will. Nearly all the muscles of the esophagus, stomach and the intestines are of this nature. They are excited to activity by the presence of food, and their movement is in no way dependent on volition.

The stomach is a pear-shaped muscular bag lined, like the mouth, with mucous membrane. It receives the food from the esophagus near the middle of the smaller or upper curve, at the largest diameter of the organ, and discharges into the intestines at its smallest end through an aperture known as the pylorus. The stomach is furnished with a number of glands which, when excited by the presence of food, secrete the fluid known as gastric juice. Pure gastric juice consists of a small quantity of saline matter in solution. It is acid owing to the presence of a small percentage of free hydrochloric acid, and contains in addition an active principle known as pepsin. This pepsin has the power of breaking up and dissolving proteid or flesh-forming matters consumed as food, such as the lean of meat, the gluten of flour, the casein of milk and cheese, the albumen of eggs, etc., and a large proportion of these substances thus dissolved is absorbed directly into the blood,

through the walls of the stomach; but the
greater bulk of the aliment, reduced to a con-

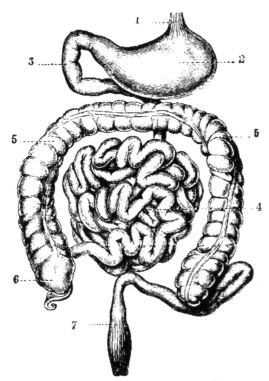

Fig. 3.—Diagram of Alimentary Tracts.

1. Lower end of esophagus.
2. Stomach.
3. Duodenum opening from pylorus.
4. Jejunum or small intestine.
5. Ascending, transverse, and descending, colon (large intestine)
6. Cæcum with vermiform appendix.
7. Rectum.

sistency resembling pea soup by the combined
action of the gastric juice, and the constant

churning produced by the muscular con-
tractions of the stomach, pass through the
pylorus into the duodenum or small intestine.
It is there mixed with the pancreatic juice,
discharged from the pancreas or sweetbread,
a strongly alkaline fluid which completes the
work of the saliva, converting that portion of
starch which has escaped the action of the
ptyalin into sugar, and emulsifying the fatty
matter of the food, reducing it to somewhat
the same state as the fat, i.e. the butter, as it
exists in milk.   It also assists the stomach in
the digestion of such proteid matters that have
left that organ insufficiently digested.   A great
deal of the digested food is taken up by vessels
called the lacteals that enter into the walls of
the small intestines, and passed into the general
circulation where it nourishes and builds up the
tissues of the body.   The digested food, nearly
deprived of its nutrient matter, passes from
the small into the large intestines where the
absorption of the surplus water and the small
remaining portion of useful constituents take
place.   The coloid or indigestible matter is
passed on to the rectum and finally discharged
from the body.   It will thus be seen that in
the mouth the amyloids or starchy matters are
acted upon, and in the stomach the proteids
are alone digested, while in the small intestine

both these, with the addition of fatty matters, are thoroughly digested, and adapted to supply the needs of the system.

Food and Nutrition.

CHEMICAL analysis shows of what substances the body is composed; and while an examination of the excretions demonstrate that all of such substances waste in greater or lesser degree, the deficiency occasioned by this waste has to be made good by the food consumed. To maintain that state of functional activity known as health, the food must contain these particular substances in such a form that the body is able to digest and assimilate them. The mineral world can supply all the elements which enter into the construction of the human body, but the system is unable to utilize them and to build up its organic constitution from non-organized elements. The plant is the alembic through which the mineral passes to adapt it to the needs of the animal economy.

From the soil, the rain and air, under the stimulus of the light and warmth of the sun, the plant builds up these complex combinations of the elementary substances that feed, sustain, and nourish the animal kingdom. Man can live and maintain his health on a diet

derived entirely from the vegetable world, or
entirely from the animal kingdom; but experience shows that in the temperate zone, at least,
a mixed diet is the most suitable.

The most perfect diet is one which gives the
whole of the required constituents of the body
in the right proportions and in an easily digestible form, and which contains a sufficient percentage of inert or indigestible matter to give it
bulk and stimulate the bowels to healthy action.
The latter ingredient is necessary, as absolutely
digestible and concentrated food stuffs produce
constipation. A man can live on wheaten flour
alone, as it contains all that is necessary to
support life, but he would starve on a diet composed of arrowroot, sugar and fat, as effectually
as he would if deprived of food altogether.

The reason of this is that while such a diet
would afford the carbon, hydrogen and oxygen
required as food, it would be totally lacking in
the nitrogen which builds up the muscles and
other tissues of the body. Vegetable foods with
few exceptions are poor in nitrogenous or flesh-
forming constituents, but rich in starch and
sugar, known as amyloids or heat and force
producers.

Nitrogen is found in the most easily digested
form in the flesh of animals; thus a properly
mixed diet affords the required proportions of

carbonaceous and nitrogenous constituents in due proportions, and the diet universally adopted in the temperate zone is economically and physiologically the most suitable to human needs.

The cereals and the pulses are comparatively rich in flesh formers, but in the latter case the nitrogen exists in the form of vegetable casein, which is difficult to digest, and probably with delicate stomachs escapes digestion altogether.

The cereals afford nitrogen as gluten, which is easily digested, but even with wheat, the most highly nitrogenized of all, the proportion of starch is considerably in excess of that required by the system. Wheaten flour as usually supplied contains 10·8 per cent of nitrogenous matter accompanied by 72·5 per cent of starchy or heat producing constituents.

A slight deficiency in the supply of certain necessary elements in the food does not necessarily mean death, but this deficiency is sure to be reflected in the health and development of the individual.

Food during Infancy in relation to the Development of the Teeth.

THE muscles, mental and nervous capabilities, the bones and teeth, all suffer from an insufficient or unsuitable diet, especially during the period of infancy. The body loses its power of resisting disease, the bones are frail, and the child becomes ricketty; the teeth are soft and deficient in their mineral constituents, and are lost early from decay. A common error is to give infants and young children a diet containing far too great an excess of starchy matter. Cornflour and arrowroot contain nothing for making bone and muscle, while very young children are quite incapable of digesting starchy foods at all. Were it not that these foods were generally prepared with milk the child would absolutely starve on them. And the nutrient value of the milk is absolutely lessened by the addition of these substances during the first ten months. Both the temporary teeth and crowns of the permanent teeth are formed during the first two years of life, and it is during this period that the most serious errors are made in the feeding that result in the lamentably faulty dentures we see in after life. The proper food during the first period of infancy is that, and that only, which has been provided by Nature for the young of mammals, viz. milk.

General observation and carefully collected statistics agree in conclusively showing that nothing can adequately replace this natural food. "The infant," says Dr. West, "whose mother refuses to perform towards it a mother's part, or who by accident, disease or death is deprived of the food that Nature destined for it, too often languishes and dies. Such children you may see with no fat to give plumpness to their limbs, no red particles in their blood to impart a healthy hue to their skin: their face wearing in infancy the lineaments of age, their voice a constant wail, their whole aspect an embodiment of woe. But give to such children the food that Nature destined for them, and if the remedy does not come too late to save them the mournful cry will cease, the face will assume a look of content; by degrees the features of infancy will disclose themselves, the limbs will grow round, the skin pure red and white, and when at length we hear the merry laugh of babyhood, it seems almost as if the little sufferer of some weeks before must have been a changeling and this the real child brought back from fairyland."

Formed for the special purpose of constituting the sole nourishment during the first period of infantile life, milk not only contains the principles required for the growth and maintenance of the body, but contains them under such a form as to be specially adapted to the feeble digestive powers then existing, which show a great want of the power of adaptiveness to alien articles of food. The teeth, which about this time begin to show themselves, indicate that preparation is now being made for the consumption of food of a solid nature, and the most suitable to begin with will be one of the farinaceous products. Bread, baked flour, biscuit powder, oatmeal, or one of the numerous kinds of nursery biscuits that are made may be employed for a time as a supplement to the previous food; then, at about the tenth month, the maternal supply, which should have been already lessened, should be altogether stopped, and the child started upon the life of independence that is to follow. For a while milk and the farinaceous products referred to above, with the addition of broth and beef tea, form a most suitable diet, but as the child advances towards its second year and the teeth become more developed, meat should be added.

Dr. W. B. Cheadle, Physician to the Hospital for Sick Children, Gt. Ormond Street, says:[1]—
" I would insist that children are naturally

---

[1] *The Book of Health* (Cassell & Co.).

animal feeders in early years. The children
fed on animal food are most robust, and that
for them to obtain perfect development they
must be supplied with a sufficient amount of it.
If milk be taken freely and well digested that
is usually sufficient; but if not, its place cannot
be supplied satisfactorily by any vegetable
material. Some other animal food such as
beef tea, meat, or eggs, is the essential substitute.

" As a matter of fact, children do not very
often suffer from any excess of animal food.
Occasionally meat given in excess disorders the
stomach or sets up gravel; but this only happens when it is taken too freely in addition to
other animal food such as milk, eggs and butter.
In truth, far greater danger lies in the other
direction. After the first year the child begins
to take bread and butter and biscuits; these
articles of food are convenient and handy: the
child likes them, and before long, perhaps,
bread and biscuit become the staple of its diet,
to the exclusion of a full proportion of animal
food. It gets bread and butter and a little
milk for breakfast, and a biscuit for luncheon;
dinner, perhaps, comprises some meat or beef
tea and pudding, while tea and supper consist
of bread with treacle or jam, or butter, and a
small quantity of milk only to drink. Thus

the child, though feeding well, grows soft in muscle, soft in bone, fragile of tooth, and backward in teething, which proves irritating, slow and painful."

It often happens, through natural causes or from the exigencies of social life, that the mother is unable to give the requisite supply of milk. In this case, next to a healthy wet nurse, a liberal supply of good cow's milk (boiled) is the best substitute; to render it more nearly identical with the human milk it should be diluted by the addition of one-third of water and a small tablespoonful of white sugar (about half-ounce) added to the pint. Later on the dilution may be diminished.

The importance of securing as far as practicable that the milk is derived from an animal in a healthy state and surrounded by wholesome conditions, will be readily understood. The alimentary canal of infants, and particularly of some, is exceedingly impressionable to unwholesome food; and the milk of cows kept, as cows in large cities and towns not unfrequently are, in an unnatural state, may prove the source of violent irritation of the stomach and bowels, and lead, if persisted in, to serious impairment of the health, terminating ultimately, it may be, in a fatal result. There can be little doubt of the desirability of always obtaining the supply from the same animal instead of indiscriminately from *any* cow, and arrangements for this are generally made in dairies.

First Dentition :

The Temporary Teeth.

MAN, of all animals the most dependent upon his own species, is not as a rule furnished with any teeth until nearer the end than the commencement of the first year of his existence, and the process has seldom terminated much before manhood is attained. During the period between birth and the possession of a sufficient number of teeth to render the individual independent of the mother, it is supplied with a food in form and composition the most suitable to its requirements, viz. a bland palatable fluid holding in solution all the constituents out of which its various tissues can be nourished and developed. Contemporaneously with the development of the teeth other organs are also becoming developed, whose function will be necessary when the former are so far advanced as to enable the individual to obtain its food from other sources, and which, being of a less simple form and character, will require more complicated processes to bring it into a condition in which it can be assimilated and turned to the same account.

This period of development is one fraught with danger to the child, as a large percentage of infant mortality can be traced directly or indirectly to the constitutional disturbances that attend dentition.

The temporary teeth in man are twenty in number—ten in the upper and ten in the lower jaw. The order and period in which they are erupted are subject to great variation.

Teeth may be erupted at or even prior to birth, or they may not appear until the second year has been completed, but in the healthy individual we may look for the lower central incisor making its appearance at the commencement of the eighth month, and being joined by its fellow a week or two later.

After an interval of two or three months the central incisors of the upper jaw appear, followed from within a month to six weeks by the lateral incisors of the same jaw.

The lower lateral incisors generally appear next in order; thus the child at the completion of its first year has eight teeth through the gums. Within another period of two months the four first molars will appear. These are erupted at the back of the jaw, leaving a space between them and the lateral incisors. At the expiration of a further four or five months this space is occupied by the canines appearing. The eruption of the second molars shortly after the second year completes the temporary set.

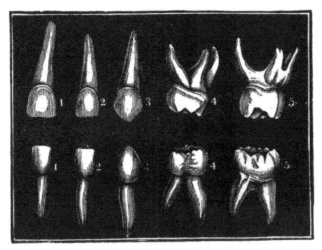

Fig. 4.—Illustrates the Temporary Teeth on the left side.

 1–1. Central incisors.
 2–2. Lateral incisors.
 3–3. Cuspids or canines.
 4–4. First or anterior molars.
 5–5. Second or posterior molar.

The order of eruption of temporary teeth is tabulated by Coleman as under—

Group.   Months.
 1. Lower central incisors **7**
   Duration of eruption one to ten days.
   Pause two to three months.

Group.   Months.

   2. Upper central and lateral incisors .   .   9

       Duration of eruption four to six weeks.

       Pause two months.

   8. Lower lateral incisors 12

      First molars 14

       Duration of eruption one to two months.

       Pause four to five months.

   4. Cuspidati (canines) 18

       Duration of eruption two to three months.

       Pause three to five months.

   5. Second molars 26

       Duration of eruption three to five months.

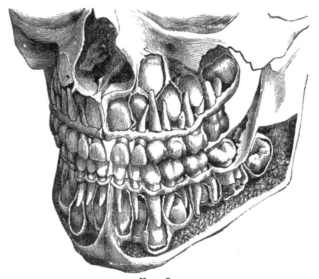

Fig. 5.

Diagram showing the two sets of teeth (temporary and permanent) in the jaws of a child of six years. Sixth-year molars are already in position, the rest of the permanent teeth in various stages of development.

Difficulties of the First Dentition.

UNDER the most favourable circumstances the teeth may appear one after another at the usual time, with so little apparent disturbance to the individual, that their presence may be only accidentally discovered.

In many cases, however, the condition of matters is not so favourable. For some time previous to the eruption of each tooth the child becomes fretful and irritable, and the gums appear hot and swollen and tender; the rubbing, evidently hitherto grateful, now causes pain and resistance.

Diarrhea, the result of intestinal irritation, is not uncommon. A troublesome cough, likewise the result of irritation conveyed to the respiratory tract, often sets in with the eruption of each tooth and, like the diarrhea, ceases when the tooth has become erupted. Eruptions are apt to appear usually on the cheek, but sometimes on the head or even over the whole body, and ulceration on the gums, lips, or on the inside of the cheeks, uneasiness and fretfulness, restless sleep or wakefulness, thirst and loss of appetite are evidences of increased constitutional disturbance, which if not relieved culminate in copious and persistent diarrhea, high fever, convulsions, and perhaps death.

Considerable relief is often afforded to the little sufferer by lancing the gum over the erupting tooth or teeth, the slight loss of blood diminishes local inflammation while the division of the tissues reduces the resistance that the tooth meets in piercing the gum. Severe constitutional symptoms frequently rapidly subside on the performance of this operation, but to be

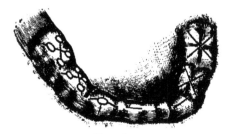

FIG. 6.
Showing direction of Incisions made in Lancing the Gum

effectual and to thoroughly relieve the tension of the gum, the cut should be made with special reference to the form of the coming tooth.

The molars require a crucial incision. In the case of either of the incisions, superior or inferior, owing to their straight edges the slightest appearance of the tooth through the gum gives entire relief so far as that particular tooth is concerned. Not so, however, with the cuspids and molars. The cuspids, it will be remembered, have cone-shaped crowns, and therefore, even after the eruption of the points, still keep up the pressure by reason of the inclosing ring of gum. A complete severance of this ring on the lateral surfaces, as well as on the anterior and posterior faces, is necessary to relieve the tension. So all the cusps or points of a molar tooth may have erupted and

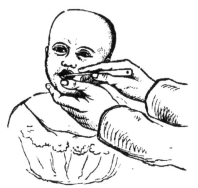

Fig. 7.—Lancing the Gum.

yet bands of gum tissue around and between them maintain a resistance as decided as before their appearance, but which is entirely over-come by cuts.

If after lancing the cuts should heal before the tooth is fairly through the gum, the opera-tion should be repeated as often as is neces-sary.

Sometimes, but not often, there is a little too much bleeding, generally caused by the child sucking the gums, incited thereto by the taste of the blood. In such case the substitution of the breast of the nurse will give the infant better employment.

The care of the Temporary Teeth.

THE temporary teeth are liable to the same causes of decay as the permanent ones, and equal care should be taken of them. It is really astonishing how little attention is generally paid to them, the prevailing idea being that as they are destined soon to be lost and give place to the second set, it is unnecessary to attempt to preserve them.

This argument as to their loss and replacement is indeed true, but other things of greater importance should be taken into consideration. The hopes of the parents are that the anticipated set will be placed evenly and beautifully in the dental arches so that no deformity may exist: that no crowded teeth will have to be extracted: that no tedious operation for regulating will be necessary, and that there may be no unusual liability to decay.

The surest way to secure the disappointment of all these commendable hopes is to be negligent in regard to the preservation of the deciduous teeth. It is not the design of Nature that the first set shall be lost by the destruction of the crowns, but by the destruction of the roots. Take care of the crowns and the roots will take care of themselves.

It is intended that simultaneously with the advance of the permanent tooth, the absorption of the root of the temporary tooth should occur, so that when the temporary tooth is thus loosened, the permanent one is generally close at hand to occupy its place. Thus no loss of space results, while it would be different if the milk teeth should be extracted months or years too soon; for any one, who has examined at all, has noticed that when a tooth has been lost and nothing has occupied the space there has been a tendency of the teeth to lean toward each other on the sides of the vacancy. Where then there is this diminution of space, it is impossible for the second teeth to arrange themselves regularly; there is barely enough room under the most favourable circumstances. Irregularly placed teeth are unusually liable to decay, both from the great difficulty of properly cleaning them, and from the fact that when such portions of enamel touch each other, as are not intended to be in antagonism, injury results. How then can the temporary teeth be preserved? The teeth should be cleaned several times daily by the parent when the child is too young to do it, and by either when the child is old enough.

The brush used should be soft and of small size. Care should be taken to cleanse the backs of the incisors and the masticating surfaces of the molars. A good tooth powder for children's use is composed of precipitated chalk, 4-ozs.; powdered orris root, 1-oz.; acid carbolic, 4 drops; oil of cassia, 2 drops; oil of rose geranium, 2 drops. The teeth should be cleansed thoroughly on rising in the morning and before retiring in the evening, but once daily is sufficiently often to use a dentifrice.

The teeth should be frequently examined by the dentist and, if decay or such imperfections in the enamel as would lead to decay should be found, the places should be filled.

If the child should be too young to undergo the more tedious operation of filling with gold, there are various fillings which are put in in a soft state and subsequently harden that preserve the teeth sufficiently well. Besides the advantages before alluded to accruing from the preservation of the deciduous teeth, it certainly is not the height of parental kindness to allow children to suffer the agonies of toothache when it can be avoided; nor is it wise to allow their early visits to a dentist to be for the purpose of having their teeth extracted, for often such a lasting unpleasant impression is made that in after years they will suffer their teeth to go to destruction rather than go near the places that are surrounded with such unpleasant associations.

Second Dentition.

Sixth-year Molar.

THE eruption of the second set begins *before* any of the first teeth are shed. Between five and a half and six and a half years of age the first permanent molars, four in number — one on each side of the upper and lower jaws— make their appearance. These are commonly supposed by parents to belong to the first set, and therefore, if found decayed shortly after their eruption, no attention is paid to them, because it is thought that they will soon have to make room for their successors, and before the error is discovered the mischief is irreparable. The sixth-year molars are the largest teeth in the mouth. In Figs. 8 and 9 they are shown in their relation to the temporary set—in a child of about six years of age. In Figs. 10 and 11 these same teeth are illustrated in their relation to the permanent set. They are very important teeth in many respects, and should never be allowed to suffer

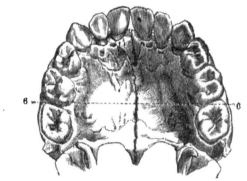

Fig. 8.—Upper Temporary Set of Teeth with **the** sixth-year Molar in position (6 6).

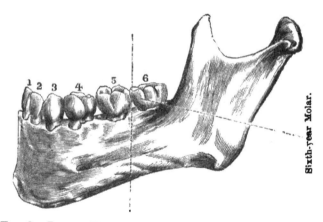

Fig. 9.—Lower Temporary Set with sixth-year Molar in position (6).

from decay if by any possibility it can be avoided. Even if they cannot be permanently

saved there are good reasons, with reference to
the preservation of the integrity of the arch,
why they should be retained up to a certain

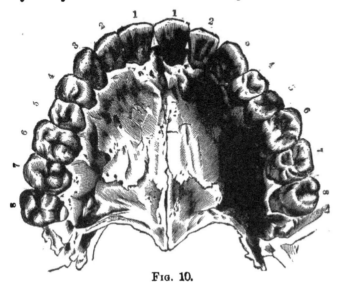

Fɪɢ. 10.

period, viz. to that between the tenth and
twelfth years—the time when the twelfth-year
molars are about to appear, and there are
equally good reasons why, if they cannot be
retained with a fair prospect of their permanent
preservation, they should be extracted at that
particular time.

Another fact which should make each one
of these teeth the object of special anxiety
on the part of the parent is that, in the
opinion of many practitioners of ripe experi-

ence, the loss of one frequently necessitates
the removal of all four in order to preserve the

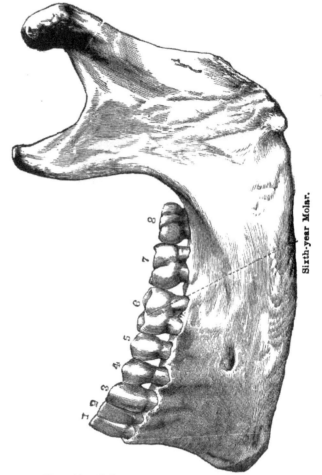

Fig. 11.—Side view of an adult lower jaw.

harmonies of articulation.   It is a good rule for
parents to count their children's teeth occasion-

ally after the fifth year, and when more than
five are found on either side of either jaw they
may know that the sixth or last one belongs to
the second or permanent set, and if lost will
never be replaced; that if extracted except at

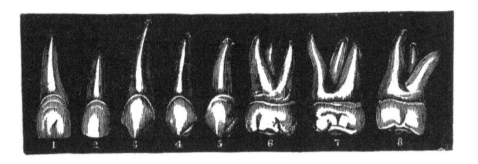

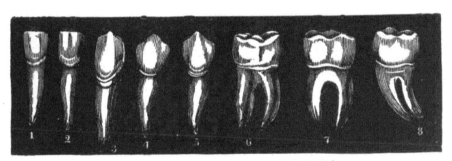

Fig. 12.—Permanent Teeth of the Left Side.

the exact time when the conditions are most
favourable, the results may be disastrous to the
entire denture, more or less interfering with
comfort and health, and by the consequent prevention of perfect mastication leading to dys-

peptic and intestinal derangements, tending to shorten life.

The want of a proper appreciation and proper treatment of these sixth-year molars is, it is safe to say, one of the most fruitful causes of the

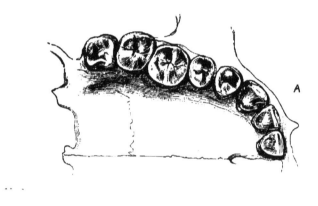

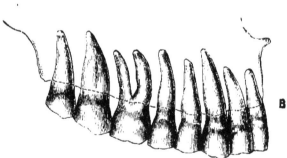

Fig. 13.—Side View and Masticating Surfaces of the Permanent Teeth. Upper Jaw.

defective masticatory apparatus of a vast majority of people at and beyond forty years of age. As the permanent teeth approach their

full development a process called absorption is
set up, by which the roots of the temporary set
are gradually removed.   Little by little the
roots are dissolved and the particles composing
them are carried away, until only the crowns

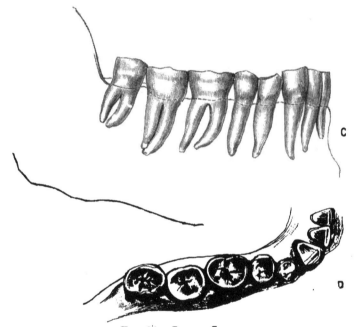

Fig. 14.—Lower Jaw.

remain. This absorptive process does not begin
upon the roots of all the temporary teeth at
once, but in the order corresponding to their
development and eruption. The lower central
incisors are the first to become loose and fall
out; then the upper central incisors : then the

laterals, and so on in the order in which they appear. Deprived of their support in the sockets, and retaining only a slight attachment to the gums, the crowns are pushed out by the movements of the tongue, cheeks or lips during mastication, or are picked out with the fingers.

The second or permanent teeth are thirty-two in number, including twelve not found in the temporary set, viz., eight bicuspids and four wisdom teeth. The following table gives the average time and order of eruption of the permanent teeth, liable however, both as to time and order, to very considerable variation in exceptional cases—

		Years.
1.	First Molars (6)	6
2. {	Central Incisors, lower jaw (1) .	7
	Central Incisors, upper jaw (1) .	8
3.	Lateral Incisors, both jaws, lower preceding upper (2). . .	9
4.	First Bicuspids (4) . . .	10
5.	Second Bicuspids (5) . . .	11
6.	Cuspidati, or Canines (3) . .	12
7.	Second Molars (7) . . .	13
8.	Third Molars (8) . . .	17 to 20

The numbers in brackets will serve to identify the form and position of these teeth by referring to Figs. 10, 11 and 12.

Troubles Attending the Second Dentition.

THE second dentition is accomplished under much more favourable conditions than the first, when the nervous apparatus is undergoing a condition of development incomparably greater than appears at any other period of life; but it occasionally happens that conditions present themselves which we must' be careful not to overlook. Thus, independently of any special symptoms, a child during the second dentition, and especially during the eruption of the molars, may appear wanting in its usual spirits, sometimes suffering, though not severely, with headache and lassitude, and the appetite is not unfrequently either diminished or capricious. Such symptoms are most commonly met with when the second molars are being erupted, and they are, though no doubt much influenced by, often attributed wholly to, the period of puberty having arrived. With a history of or tendency to epilepsy the period of the second dentition is one of importance and anxiety, especially during that of the eruption of the third molars, and a considerable increase in the number and frequency of the fits often occurs, followed generally by an improvement upon the complete eruption of the teeth.

D

The local symptoms attending the second dentition are also generally less severe than with the first, but it is by no means uncommon to find the mouth so swollen that the gums of the upper and lower jaws over the erupting teeth come in contact before the remainder of the teeth meet rendering the complete closing of the jaws impossible, and any attempt at mastication futile and painful. Soothing applications to the gum such as an infusion of poppyheads will usually result in the rapid subsidence of the swelling, or if the mouth is hot and painful and the gum white and tense, manifestly stretched over the crown of the tooth, the employment of the lancet will soon give relief. With the eruption of the third molars, or wisdom teeth, as they are called, considerable trouble is often experienced. Those in the lower jaw especially often appear so far back that only one cusp or point shows through the gum, the rest of the crown being buried in the folds of soft flesh that connect the upper and lower jaws at the back of the mouth. This flesh is not attached to the crown of the tooth, as can readily be ascertained by a probe, but forms a sac or bag enclosing it. This sac is not self cleansing, and is liable to become offensive, owing to the imprisonment of the secretions, or from other causes giving rise to swelling and severe inflammatory symptoms which, spreading to the muscles, either impede or totally prevent the movement of the jaw (trismus). A complete removal of the membrane covering the top of the tooth either by the lancet or gum scissors, afterwards fomenting the part with hot infusion of poppyheads, to which a small quantity of chlorate of potash has been added, is the treatment usually successful. A recurrence of the trouble may take place, as the gum sometimes slowly creeps back and again partly covers the crown, and the extraction either of the second molar, if decayed, or of the imperfectly erupted wisdom tooth will prove the only effectual remedy.

Irregularity of the Teeth.

IRREGULARITY is more common with the second than with the first set, and it is always more important, as the defect lasts through life.

The symmetrical appearance of the teeth and their utility for mastication depend to a great extent on their occupying their regular places in the dental arches. In the normal mouth the points or cusps of the back teeth in the lower jaw fit into the depressions of those in the upper jaw, thus presenting the greatest possible surface for mastication. Irregularity of position by interfering with this perfect occlusion greatly reduces the masticating efficacy of the teeth, while the impossibility of cleaning the spaces between crowded and irregular teeth is favourable to their early destruction by decay. Pronunciation is often rendered indistinct and the lips, gums, and tongue irritated by teeth projecting inside or outside the dental arch. The deviation from the normal position may vary both in form and extent. Simply one tooth may be slightly displaced, or the whole set may be in such an indescribable state of confusion that scarcely a single tooth seems to occupy the place properly assigned to it, seriously interfering with the symmetry of the face and the mastication of the food.

Irregularity may arise from a variety of causes—from the too early removal or from the undue retention of the temporary teeth : from a disparity in size between the jaws and the teeth, large teeth being erupted in a small jaw or, vice versâ, through injuries to the jaw during the development of the teeth : from the presence of extra or supernumerary teeth : from a persistent indulgence in such habits as sucking the tongue, fingers, or thumb during childhood. The habitually open mouth, continually associated with enlarged tonsils and mouth breathing, also tends to produce a contracted and ill-developed V-shaped dental arch furnished with crowded and irregular teeth.

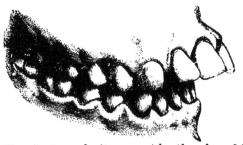

Fig. 15.—An irregularity caused by thumb sucking.

The V-shaped, contracted dental arch is quite amenable to treatment and is generally expanded by the use of a plate fitting the palate with or without covering the teeth. The plate is sawn in half and a spring is introduced, in such a manner that it has a constant tendency to force the two halves apart.

Disproportion in size of the upper and lower jaws is of frequent occurrence. The upper teeth are often very short and much too far outside the lower ones so that the front teeth actually rest on the lower lip, completely hiding the lower teeth, when the jaws are closed. Frequently the cutting edges of the upper teeth shut squarely on those of the lower, causing both to wear away.

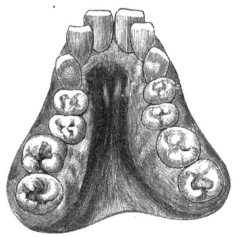

Fig. 16.—Upper jaw with contracted V-shaped dental arch.

In other instances the lower jaw protrudes and the teeth are thrown far in advance of the

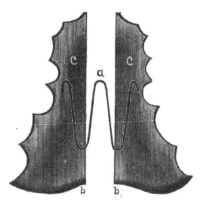

Fig. 17.—Split plate with spring (a) for expanding dental arch.

upper ones, giving a "bull-dog" appearance
that is anything but agreeable. Occasionally
the back teeth alone antagonize, while there
remains a considerable space between the front
teeth which cannot be closed by any effort.

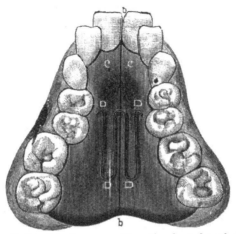

Fig. 18.—Split plate for expanding the dental arch in position
in the mouth.

The incisors, canines, and bicuspids are
frequently seen to have a portion of their
number crowded outside the arch, while
others are pushed inside, some of the teeth
of the opposite jaw shutting among them in
such a way as to lock them in their irregular
positions.

The same teeth are often turned partially
around, lapping over one another, or having
their sides presented where the fronts ought

to be. In some cases the teeth change places,
the canine exchanging position with the
lateral, or the lateral with the central, etc.
The failure of certain teeth to erupt, after the
loss of the temporary ones, allows their un-
filled spaces to be encroached upon by the

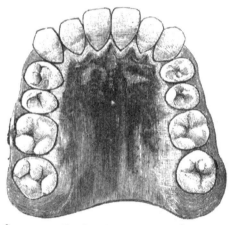

Fig. 19.—Same mouth after treatment with spring expanding
plate showing a great improvement in conformation of the dental
arch.

neighbouring teeth, causing a straggling appearance.

The same condition often occurs from the
loss of teeth by decay or accident where there
is no artificial substitute. Teeth sometimes
erupt in the roof of the mouth and deformed
and supernumerary teeth appear in different
parts of the arch.

Figs. 20 to 22 illustrate the evil results of

the too early removal of the temporary canine teeth.

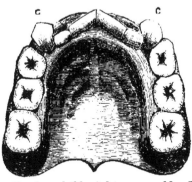

F<small>IG</small>. 20.—Mouth of a child eight years old. The four front permanent teeth are compelled to assume an irregular position owing to the small size of the jaw.

Fig. 20 shows the mouth of a child about eight years of age. It frequently happens, as in this case, that the four permanent front

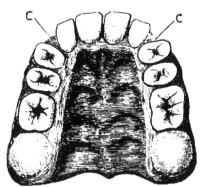

F<small>IG</small>. 21.—Same mouth as fig. 20 at eleven years of age. The temporary canines c c fig. 20 having been improperly extracted to give room to the four front teeth. The teeth have thus been allowed to occupy the space required for the permanent canines (fig. 21, c c).

teeth appear in the space previously occupied by the same number of small temporary teeth, and consequently are forced to assume a more

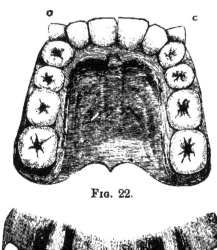

FIG. 22.

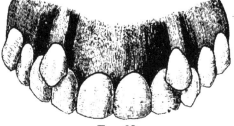

FIG. 23.

FIGS. 22 and 23 show the same mouth as fig. 20 at the age of fourteen. The too early extraction of the temporary canines has prevented the normal growth of the jaw, and thus no room remains for the permanent canines which are erupted outside the arch.

or less irregular position. Now obviously the easiest way to give room for the newly erupted permanent teeth to arrange themselves regularly is to extract the temporary canines (fig. 20, c c). The immediate result of such treatment is very satisfactory and by the eleventh year the teeth have assumed the position shown in fig. 21. About the completion of the twelfth year the permanent canines are erupted. As there is no space remaining for them they are forced outside the arch as shown in figs. 22, 23, and produce an unsightly irregularity and one extremely difficult to treat successfully.

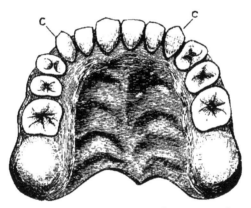

Fig. 24.—Shows probable condition of same mouth as fig. 20 at the age of eleven, no teeth having been extracted, the four front irregular teeth having assumed a regular position through the room afforded by the natural growth of the jaw. c c are the *temporary* canines, the rest of the teeth belong to the permanent set.

Returning to fig. 20, if the temporary canines (c c) had been allowed to remain, the natural growth of the jaw would have allowed the irregular front permanent teeth to assume the normal position without the extraction of the temporary canines (fig. 20, c c) in the course of a year or so, and by the end of the eleventh year the teeth would have been equally

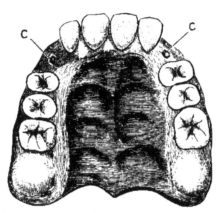

FIG. 25.—Same mouth as fig. 24 at the age of thirteen. The temporary canines have been shed leaving ample room for their permanent successors which are just appearing through the gum at c c.

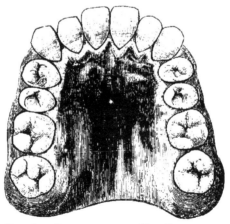

Fig. 26.—Showing the same case after the permanent canines have been erupted, all the teeth being regular.

regular, and a better development of the jaw
would have resulted from the retention of the
temporary canines (fig. 24, c c), while those
teeth would have preserved the place for the
reception of the permanent canines when the
time for their appearance was reached as
shown by fig. 25.

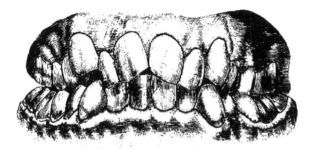

Fig. 27.—A case of irregularity.

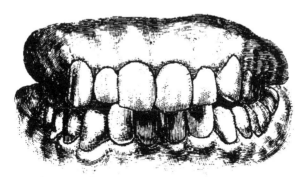

Fig. 28.—The same mouth after treatment.

Judicious extraction to give room, filing,
plates, ligatures, screws, caps, inclined planes,
etc., are the means generally employed to

correct irregularities; but it will be impossible
to lay down any directions which will be appli-
cable to all cases, as there are hardly any two
precisely alike. It may be received as a general
truth, however, that any case of irregularity
of the teeth can be either completely corrected,
or very materially improved by use of the

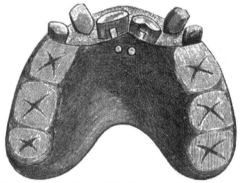

Fig. 29.—Upper regulating plate in mouth, plate covering back
teeth.

proper means. The patient should be neither
too young nor too old. If too young the subsequent changes of the growing jaws may operate
against permanent benefit; and a lack of the
appreciation of the good results would prevent
the diligence demanded from the patient in
wearing the appliances, keeping them cleaned,
etc. If too old the teeth are so firmly set that
it requires a much greater amount of time in
which to accomplish a certain result.

For anything like a complicated case, from twelve to fifteen years of age is the best time. Slight irregularities, such as two teeth presenting anteriorly or posteriorly, may be treated much earlier.

Fig. 29 represents a type of case where very early treatment is imperative; it illustrates an

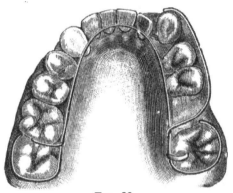

FIG. 30.

upper jaw in which the two central incisors have erupted in the palate, with their cutting edges inside the lower teeth. As the lower teeth bite outside them when the mouth is closed they cannot possibly move forward without the aid of a mechanical appliance. The regulating plate is shown *in situ*. It is necessary to cover the back teeth in order to allow the upper front teeth to pass in free of the lowers. Mastication is carried cn by the lower back teeth biting on the regulating plate. The irregular incisors are forced forward by small pegs of compressed hickory, which swelling by the absorption of the moisture in the mouth, gradually force the irregular teeth forward. These pegs have frequently to be renewed.

Fig. 30 represents a lower jaw with a wire spring regulating appliance in its place, de-

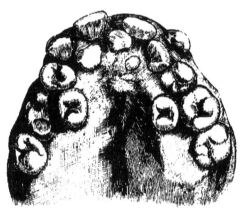

Fig. 31.

signed to retract a canine tooth which has come through the gum too far forward.

The regulation of teeth frequently requires great patience both on the part of the patient and the operator. The appliance has to be worn for many months, and frequent alterations of the springs, wires and ligatures are necessary. Trouble sometimes arises owing to the visits to the dentist interfering with the school attendance, and the treatment of a case is often rendered protracted and unsatisfactory by the dentist having to regulate his appointments by the holidays of his patient rather than by the exigencies of the case.

After the teeth have been directed into the required position, it is often still necessary to wear the plate for some months until the teeth become consolidated into their new position.

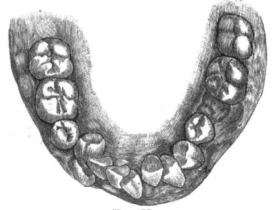

Fig. 32.

Much can be done in even the most hopeless looking cases of irregularity of the teeth. Figs. 31 and 32 are drawn from the models of an extremely complicated case of dental irregularity which came under the care of a well-known practitioner.

E

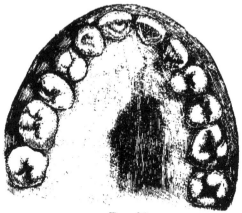

FIG. 33.

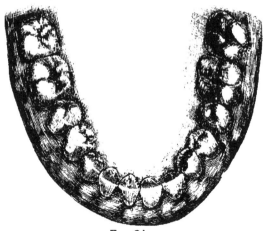

FIG. 34.

Figs. 33 and 34 show the same mouth after treatment extending over a period of two years.

The successful result here shown could only

be obtained where the dentist's efforts are seconded by a thorough co-operation on the part of the patient.

The Structure of the Teeth.

THE structure and composition of the teeth present many points of interest, and help to enlighten us in acquiring a knowledge necessary to promote their welfare. The portion of the tooth visible as it occupies its natural position in the mouth is known as the crown; that portion concealed by the gum is known as the root, while the line at which the gum first comes in contact with the tooth is called the neck. The roots of the teeth are fixed in sockets of thin bone, which are formed simultaneously with them, and are known as alveoli, and by which they are firmly embraced. The bulk of the tooth is built up of an ivory-like substance known as dentine. The crown is covered and protected by a thin layer of enamel, which is a tissue of extraordinary hardness. The root is covered with a similar layer of different structure known as cementum. In the centre of the tooth is a cavity containing the pulp, or as it is popularly known, as the nerve of the tooth. This pulp is a wormlike fleshy structure containing a nerve, vein and artery, and assists in the formation and nutrition of the tooth. The position of these tissues can be seen from the accompanying illustration (fig. 35), which represents a molar split vertically and transversely to show the relative positions occupied by the various tissues composing it.

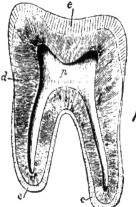

The enamel is the cap or covering of the crown : it is the hardest tissue of the body. It is thickest on the cutting edges and masticating surfaces, gradually becoming thinner towards the neck, at which point it is met or slightly overlapped by the cementum. The enamel is possessed of very slight, if of any, sensibility. It contains not more than four per cent of animal matter, and is almost entirely soluble in acids. Under the microscope it is found to consist of rows of hexagonal parallel fibres lying side by side.

Fig. 35.

a, Longitudinal Section of a Molar.

b, Transverse Section.
(c) The cementum.
(d) The dentine.
(e) The enamel.
(n) The pulp or nerve of the tooth.

The cementum is a layer of hard tissue covering the roots of the teeth. It is intermediate in hardness between dentine and bone, resembling the latter more than either of the other hard tissues found in a tooth. It is thickest at the end of the root, gradually diminishing until it seems to unite with or slightly overlap the enamel at the neck of the tooth. The dentine or so-called ivory constitutes the bulk of the tooth. It is, so to speak, its framework, giving each tooth its size and shape. If the enamel and cementum were removed the dentine would still preserve the general form of the tooth. It contains over one-fourth of animal matter, and when subjected to the action of acids the earthy matter is dissolved out, leaving a cartilage-like mass retaining the form of the tooth. Examined microscopically it is found to consist of innumerable tubes of a diameter of about $\frac{1}{1800}$ of an inch. It is usually highly sensitive both to variations of temperature and to contact with foreign substances. It owes its sensitiveness to the pulp of the tooth, and when the pulp dies the dentine loses its sensibility.

Decay of the Teeth.

CARIES, or dental decay, is one of the most prevalent diseases of modern life, and it evinces so strong a tendency to increase that it is rare to find an individual among the civilized portions of the human race whose mouth does not show some evidence of its ravages, or who has never experienced the pain that accompanies it.

The causes of decay are predisposing and exciting. The predisposing causes are imperfect structure, irregularity of position, and mechanical injuries. Conditions inherent in the teeth by virtue of their original structure determined before birth or during infancy, establish in many cases a predisposition to decay.

Owing either to imperfect health of the mother during the development of the teeth, or to disturbances of the health of the child during their formative stage, the various processes of organization are liable to be so interrupted and deranged as to result in defective dental structures. The dentine is soft and friable, the enamel semi-crystallized and deficient in quantity and quality—a heterogenous mixture of animal and earthy materials. Teeth thus imperfect in their texture are necessarily not fitted to resist the action of destructive agents.

The same may be said of those with deep fissures, reaching through the enamel to the dentine, whose edges are imperfectly joined.

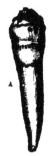

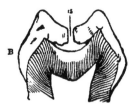

Fig. 86.—B. Section of a Molar showing a fault or fissure in the enamel (*a*) caused by imperfect development. These fissures are frequently the starting point of decay.

Fig. 86.—A. Upper Canine Tooth with badly formed enamel.

Neglect of the temporary teeth is a pregnant cause of the decay of the permanent set. The process of shedding the temporary teeth extends over a period of six years. Under normal conditions the appearance of its permanent successor is simultaneous with the falling out of the temporary tooth, and owing to the order in which the temporary teeth are shed temporary and permanent teeth stand side by side in the same mouth, in certain positions, for several years.

The permanent lateral incisor is erupted during the eighth year: the temporary canine is not lost until the thirteenth year, and thus

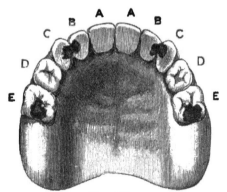

FIG. 37.

Figs. 37–39 are intended to illustrate the disastrous effect of decayed temporary teeth on the permanent set. The temporary teeth are distinguished in the cuts by the letters A, B, C, D, E; the permanent teeth by the numbers 1, 2, 3, 4, 5, 6, 7, 8.

Fig. 37 shows the Upper Jaw of a child five years of age, the temporary lateral incisors (B B), the canines (C C), and the posterior molars (E E) are decayed.

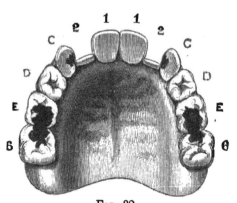

FIG. 38.

Fig. 38 shows the same mouth during the eighth year; the permanent centrals (1 1) have appeared and the laterals (2 2) are being erupted in close contact with the temporary canines (C C). The two permanent molars (6 6) have been in position some time and have become carious through contact with the second temporary molars (E E).

these teeth remain in close contiguity to each other for a period of four years. The first permanent molar makes its appearance during the sixth year, and from that time until the twelfth year remains in contact with the second temporary molar.

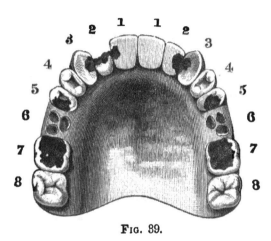

Fig. 89.

Fig. 39 represents the same mouth at the age of nineteen. The left lateral (2), originally rendered carious by contact with decayed temporary canine (fig. 88, c), has broken off and rendered the permanent canine (B) and central (1) carious, while on the right side the decay originating in the temporary canine (figs. 87 and 88, c c) has effected the permanent lateral (2), and through that tooth the permanent canine (3). The first permanent molar each side has decayed away to a mere stump, causing the second permanent molar (7 7) and the posterior bicuspid (5 5) to decay. Thus, at the age of nineteen, eleven teeth of the permanent set are rendered useless, as the direct result of the neglect of the decayed temporary canines and molars in the mouth at the age of five years.

Now if the temporary canine happens to be decayed the caries rapidly spreads to the permanent lateral incisor, while the decayed temporary molar communicates the disease to the first permanent molar. The germs of decay are thus conducted from the first to the second set of teeth, and the decay spreads from one to another until every tooth in the mouth is in a ruinous and useless condition, possibly before the sufferer is out of his teens.

Mr. Chas. S. Tomes points out that : " In a perfectly normal, well-formed jaw the teeth are individually so shaped, and are so arranged that they touch one another by curved surfaces only, so that the areas of contact are very small.

"As teeth are not rigidly fixed, but are capable of a small degree of motion, they rub against their neighbours, and in time wear the curved surfaces of contact into small flat facets, but still the areas of contact remain small, and are well removed from the gum.

" But in a crowded mouth this is all altered ; the teeth standing irregularly come into contact with their neighbours by other than the proper surfaces, and oftentimes they touch over a far larger area, extending right down to the gums. And when the oft - repeated slight motions of the tooth begin to take effect, enamel is crushed or worn away over irregular areas which, damaged thus, as well as by being lurking places for fermentation to go on in, become the starting points of decay."

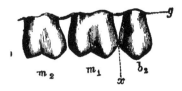

Fig. 40.—The second Bicuspid and first and second Molar teeth, showing the surfaces in contact (*x*) are very small; *g*, edge of gum.

Irregularity of position, from whatever cause, renders the teeth liable to decay.

When they lap over one another or touch at points other than those which are intended to come in contact in a natural and orderly arrangement, decay at such points is apt to occur.

The difficulty of keeping irregular teeth clean is another fruitful cause of decay, the retention of food being favoured by their positions. Mechanical injuries—falls, blows, and improper use of the teeth, destroying the continuity of the enamel—also predispose to decay.

The exciting causes of decay are chiefly different forms of chemical action, which may either follow from the use of acids as food or medicine, or be caused by improper tooth-powders or washes; or may result from a vitiation of the secretions of the mouth, either from a general systematic derangement, or from a local cause, such as mumps, sore throat, or the presence of tartar about the necks of the teeth, causing an irritation of the gums and inducing an acid secretion; or from the fermentation and decomposition of food about and between the teeth.

Decay never begins on the smooth surfaces of teeth—those which are exposed to the friction of mastication—but always commences at points which, owing to their structure and arrangement, furnish convenient receptacles for decay-producing agents. The points most favourable to such retention are the deep fissures of the bicuspids and molars (fig. 36B), and the sides of the teeth where they come in contact with each other. In these crevices and at the surfaces which the teeth present to each other, and which favour the lodgment and retention of food and mucus, decay is most likely to begin and, once begun, to continue. It proceeds slowly, perhaps, so far as the enamel is concerned, but when it reaches the dentine, either through a fissure in the enamel, or a breach made through its walls, it progresses more rapidly until the pulp is reached, and its vitality and the strength and substance of the tooth are destroyed.

Whatever may be said of the deleterious effects of tobacco upon the general system, it has not been proved to have any influence in the production of caries, although the discoloration which results from its continued use detracts markedly from the appearance of the teeth.

Sugar and confections exercise no directly injurious effects upon the teeth, but when taken in excess produce an acid condition of the stomach, unfavourable to the health of the mouth, and when left in the interstices of the teeth rapidly undergo an acid fermentation, resulting in a product capable of acting very injuriously upon tooth structure.

The process of decay of the teeth is as varied in different individuals and at different times as is the character of the disintegration. It proceeds sometimes insidiously and slowly, and again with wonderful rapidity, sometimes announcing its ravages by a sensitiveness of the exposed dentine to sweets and acids and to changes of temperature, and at other times giving no notice of its presence until an exposure of the pulp has been made, when the pangs of toothache are experienced.

Toothache and Neuralgia.

When from exposure by decay or other causes the pulp becomes irritated and inflamed, the pain known as toothache arises; but during the progress of decay, even before the exposure of the pulp has been effected, pain of more or less severity may be experienced, frequently diffused over the sides and top of the head, and not apparently referable to the teeth at all.

These pains are generally ascribed to neuralgia even by medical practitioners, and quinine and other tonics are prescribed and taken in considerable quantities, without effect. After a course of medical attendance the patient is referred to the dentist and a careful examination of the mouth frequently reveals several unsuspected cavities, the treatment of which gives immediate relief from suffering.

When consulted in cases of neuralgic pains about the head and neck it is advisable in most cases for the medical man to refer his patient to the dentist for a thorough examination of the mouth as a preliminary to treatment, and not to delay doing so until the failure of medicine to alleviate the pain points conclusively to the fact that the trouble is of dental origin.

It is true that the physician looks at the

teeth before prescribing, but many teeth that appear sound on a mere inspection of the mouth prove to be badly decayed when thoroughly examined by a dental surgeon, who, by aid of his special appliances and knowledge, is better able to diagnose defects in the teeth than the general medical practitioner.

Dr. W. H. Williamson, in his presidential address to the Aberdeen Medico-Chirurgical Society on the relation of Dentistry to Medical Education, remarking on the subject, says :—

" Take, for example, the simple, but yet very important point of the examination of the teeth, not unfrequently attempted by doctors for the purpose of ascertaining the cause of facial neuralgia, which in ninety-nine cases out of a hundred is of dental origin. A general glance of the opened mouth is taken, and if there is no blackness or distinct hole to be seen the verdict is that, as the teeth seem sound, therefore they may be excluded from the list of causes. This superficial idea of what constitutes an examination leads to many errors of diagnosis.

"Very early in practice I remember a case of a lady who had been under the care of a very deservedly celebrated London consultant, who is cited in one of our dental books as having been remarkably acute in diagnosing obscure cases of dental disease. The patient was suffering from neuralgia, and her mouth was in due course examined, but as no cause was discovered there she was put on a course of some anti-neuralgic, which did her no good. It would seem just at first sight, when she opened her mouth, that it was a very simple matter to tell whether her teeth were the source of trouble or not, for on the affected side—on the lower jaw at any rate—there was but one solitary molar coming well forward which had quite a good, sound-looking appearance, but on pressing the cheek away with the finger a large cavity was disclosed on the outside, with an exposed pulp at the bottom of it. The destruction of the pulp cured in a couple of hours a painful affection of some two months' standing.

It is only during the past two or three years that the medical profession has generally recognized the potent influence of defective teeth as a factor in the production of systematic disease. Attention was attracted to this subject by a most convincing paper read by Mr. J. F. Colyer at the General Meeting of the British Dental Association, in 1902, which clearly traced the disastrous effect of decayed and neglected teeth on the system, and he supported his position by bringing forward many instances in which the most intractable diseases of the nerves, blood, stomach, and intestines progressed towards a cure directly the teeth had been put in proper order.

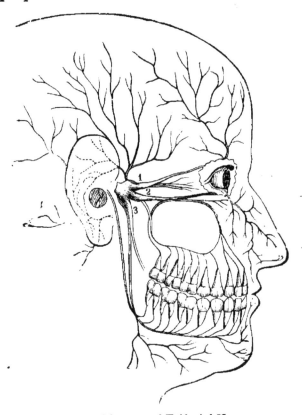

Fig. 41.—Diagram of Trifacial Nerves.

1, Ophthalmic branch.
2, Superior maxillary branch (upper jaw).
3, Inferior maxillary branch (lower jaw).

Neuralgic pains of dental origin are due to reflected or sympathetic action. It will be seen

F

by referring to the diagram of the nervous con-
nections of the teeth that they consist of three
main branches which ramify to almost every
part of the face, mouth and head, and irritation
to one branch often gives rise to pain at a
portion of the nerve very remote from the
source of injury. Thus the irritation caused
by a decayed tooth in the lower jaw may be
reflected in such a manner that the pain is
experienced in the upper jaw, and vice versâ.

Toothache arising from the Inflammation of the Nerve of the Tooth (Pulpitis).

The occurrence of pain in a tooth is generally evidence of the exposure and consequent
inflammation of the nerve.   It is then necessary
to kill the nerve (or pulp) and afterwards
remove it and to fill the pulp cavity with an
antiseptic stopping, and finally to stop the
cavity caused by decay.   When the nerve has
been thus killed the tooth is what is technically
known as "dead," and although a tooth in
this condition may remain useful for years
there is a liability for it to become loose,
tender, and ultimately abscessed, necessitating
its removal.

In the past terrible sufferings were inflicted

on unhappy patients in attempts to destroy the nerve of a tooth by hot needles, etc. But the operation, as now performed, is quite painless. The decayed dentine is cleared away as far as possible, a small portion of specially prepared paste placed in contact with the exposed nerve and a temporary stopping inserted in the tooth. This is allowed to remain from twenty-four to forty-eight hours.

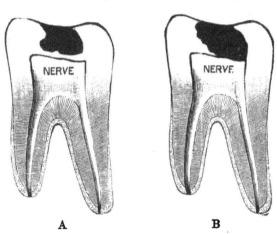

A   B

Fig. 42.—Sections of decayed teeth showing (A) tooth in which the decay has not reached the pulp cavity (or nerve), and which can be therefore stopped without destroying the pulp. B Tooth in which the decay has reached the pulp cavity (or nerve), and destruction of the pulp is necessary.

On taking out this stopping the nerve is found quite dead and has then to be removed from the tooth and the pulp cavity filled and the tooth stopped.

Considerable misapprehension exists in the

public mind with regard to "killing the nerve," and it is not unusual for a patient with an aching tooth and swollen face to request the dentist to "kill the nerve" of the tooth, perfectly oblivious to the fact that the trouble is really an abscess set up by the dead and decomposed nerve.   When the sufferer is informed that the nerve is already dead he looks incredulous and assures the dentist that he (the dentist) is mistaken.   "The tooth aches.   How can a tooth ache if the nerve is dead?"   The pain in a dead tooth arises from inflammation of the membrane lining the socket of the tooth and is distinguished from pulpitis (i.e. tooth-ache arising from inflammation of the nerve) by the tooth feeling longer than usual and preventing the patient closing the mouth with comfort, and is frequently accompanied by swelling.   With pulpitis no swelling occurs, and the teeth coming into contact on closing the mouth cause no uneasiness.

Killing the nerve or pulp is only a pre-liminary to filling the tooth, and unless followed up by stopping would in the majority of cases be injurious rather than beneficial in its results and lead to the production of an abscess at the root of the tooth.

For the relief of toothache arising from ex-posure of the pulp (pulpitis), a little ball of cotton wool saturated with oil of cloves or carbolized collodion perhaps is the best amateur treatment. Care must be taken not to smear either of these agents over the lips or face, as they will cause painful blisters. When once a tooth has ached a recurrence of the trouble is likely, and permanent relief can only be obtained by consulting a dentist and having the tooth properly stopped or, if necessary, extracted.

Periodontitis and Alveolar Abscess (Gum-boil).

ALTHOUGH the complete or proximate exposure of the pulp and its consequent inflammation (pulpitis) is one of the most frequent causes of toothache, this pain may arise from other sources. The sockets of the teeth are lined by a delicate membrane, attached both to alveoli or sockets and to the cementum of the tooth. This membrane may become inflamed and thickened, lifting the tooth slightly in its socket, and making it feel long and tender, rendering mastication difficult; until as the inflammatory action increases, it becomes impossible to close the mouth without experiencing intense pain. This form of toothache known as periodontitis is often amenable to treatment, but if neglected generally culminates in gum-boil or alveolar abscess, and occasionally in the necrosis or death of a portion of the jaw bone.

Periodontitis may arise from cold, mechanical injury, or the accumulation of tartar round the necks of the teeth, but the most severe cases are generally those associated with "dead teeth," that is, teeth in which the nerve has died through exposure by decay, broken down teeth and roots, which, after giving pain, have ceased to ache for some time.

The nerve canals of such teeth are generally in an indescribably foul condition owing to the putrifaction of the dead pulp, and filled with highly septic matter, a particle of which, accidentally forced through the opening at the point of the root, by which the nerve originally entered the tooth is quite sufficient to set up violent inflammation in the socket of the tooth, often accompanied by severe constitutional symptoms, swelling of the face and neck, and abscess at the root of the tooth, the resulting pus generally finds its way to the surface of the gum opposite the abscess, or at some other point in the mouth, forming what is popularly known as "gum-boil." After the discharge of the pus the pain subsides and the swelling gradually disappears.

But the disease is not cured, and after a longer or shorter period, depending on various circumstances—notably on the good or ill health of the individual—there will be a recurrence of the abscess. If this is repeated too often the bony socket of the tooth becomes affected, the sockets of adjoining teeth participate in the trouble, the teeth lose their vitality and drop out, and sometimes necrosis (death) of a portion of the jaw follows. Sometimes the pus instead of finding exit near the affected tooth, burrows among the tissues, and makes an outlet for itself at a distant point inside or outside of the mouth, not infrequently producing disfiguring scars on the face. When the symptoms indicate periodontitis treatment should be instituted with a view to prevent the formation of an abscess, or if this effort fails, to influence it to open at a desirable point— inside of the mouth and not upon the face.

Domestic treatment is usually wrongly directed, and that prescribed by the average general practitioner is equally at fault. The best possible advice that can be given is to consult a dental surgeon at an early stage of the trouble, at which time it can frequently be averted.

The treatment of alveolar abscess is within the province of the dental surgeon, and his experience and facilities for the antiseptic treatment of teeth and other necessary opera-

tions in the reduction of alveolar abscess are
greater than those of the family medical man.
If unable to consult a dentist immediately, an
excellent palliative treatment is fomenting the

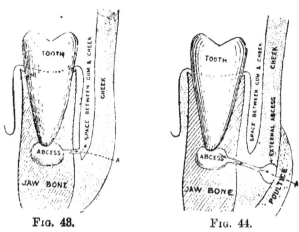

FIG. 43.   FIG. 44.

Fig. 43 shows a section of the lower jaw with a tooth having
an abscess under it which, by treatment such as hot fomenta-
tions used inside the mouth, has been led to discharge into the
space existing between the cheek and the gum, causing no disfigurement.

Fig. 44 represents what would probably occur if the same
abscess were treated by poulticing the outside of the face. The
pus being drawn towards the poultice would discharge through
the cheek forming an ugly and permanent scar.

inside of the mouth with hot water or with an
infusion of poppy heads (made by boiling 2 ozs.
of poppy heads for ten minutes in a pint of
water) held in the mouth, or a toasted fig held
against the gum will frequently give great
relief and hasten the forming of the abscess. A
poultice should *never* be used on the *outside* of the

face, and if the extraction is necessary, it is *not advisable to wait until the swelling subsides*, but

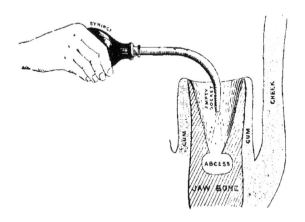

Fig. 45.

Fig. 45 explains the treatment of alveolar abscess by the extraction of the tooth causing it. The abscess sac is broken by the extraction, and the pus can be removed by syringing well with a weak solution of carbolic acid or Listerine.

to have the tooth out at the *earliest possible moment*. The extraction is almost invariably followed by a complete evacuation of the abscess and a subsidence of inflammatory symptoms.

As the alveolar abscess forms it dissolves or absorbs a portion of the bone of the jaw, thus forming a cavity at the bottom of the socket which is occupied by the abscess sac, a membraneous bag containing pus.

The following typical case of a disfiguring external wound on the face, caused by improper treatment of an alveolar abscess, is given by the dental surgeon to the Evelina Hospital for Sick Children—

"A. F., a girl aged five years, of pallid complexion, complains of a sore on her face. Had toothache some months ago; three weeks since the face suddenly swelled up, causing much pain. It was well poulticed by the mother. The child had an unhealthy-looking sore on the left cheek opposite the molar region of the lower jaw. It was small in size, circumscribed, and on its summit there was a small papilla from which pus was oozing. Careful probing showed a direct connexion with the roots of a lower temporary molar which was found deeply carious, but firm in its socket. This was removed and in one week the scar alone remained."

This gentleman, commenting on this case, writes: "As in this instance advice is often sought when the mischief is done." It also illustrates a method of treatment frequently adopted by the ignorant, viz., that of poulticing swellings upon the face which, if nothing else happens, may leave a life-long scar.

Dr. W. H. Williamson, in his presidential address to the Aberdeen Medico-Chirurgical

Society, January, 1901, on " The Relation of Dentistry to Medical Education," says :

" When an alveolar abscess is developing it is by no means an uncommon error for a doctor

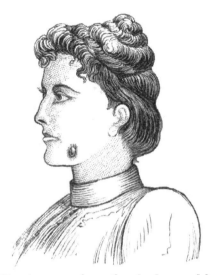

Fɪɢ. 46.—Showing wound on the cheek caused by poulticing an alveolar abscess (gum-boil).

to advise outside poulticing, the consequence being external fistula, leaving more or less of a scar on the face, according to the length of time it has been allowed to remain untreated ; that is to say, the offending tooth or root not having been removed. When this however is done, it is astonishing with what rapidity the sinus heals up without any further treatment whatever."

In practice cases are often met with where medical men have directed poulticing the face for alveolar abscess and have afterwards lanced the abscess on the exterior of the cheek or under the chin, producing an unsightly scar. Under *dental* treatment an external wound from an abscessed tooth is practically unknown. Even when the pus is on the point of discharging through the cheek the dentist strengthens the skin by painting with collodion, supports it with a bandage and opens and disperses the contents of the abscess either through the socket or by lancing the *inside* of the mouth, thus avoiding all risk of disfigurement.

Stopping or Filling the Teeth.

THE process of removing the diseased portion of the tooth and replacing the loss by a substitute is known as stopping or filling—this is one of the most useful operations in dentistry, and when resorted to in time will almost invariably preserve a tooth and render it useful for a considerable period. Many, through a most unaccountable prejudice, will allow their teeth to decay one by one, enduring all the pain and misery attending a diseased and neglected mouth, rather than submit to the operation of filling, although in by far the greater proportion of cases it is perfectly painless, especially when professional aid is resorted to in an early stage of the disease, and when the best result can be attained.

The true advantages of filling are unknown to those who only consult the dentist when driven to do so by pain. An aching tooth can, after treatment, be successfully stopped, but the probability of success is far less than in cases where the stopping is completed before the exposure of the nerve, when the tooth needs no preliminary treatment except the removal of the decayed and softened tissue.

The materials used for stopping are numerous, and range from gold to gutta percha. Gold is certainly the best and most durable stopping in suitable teeth, but in frail and rapidly decaying soft teeth it frequently proves very unsatisfactory, while with nervous and timid patients the strain of having a large gold filling inserted and consolidated is more than they can readily endure.

In these cases plastic fillings are employed. Plastic fillings consist of (*a*) Amalgams, (*b*) Osteo or cement fillings, (*c*) Gutta percha. Amalgams consist of a combination of gold, platinum, tin, silver and other metals, with a small proportion of quicksilver, and are introduced into the cavity in a pasty condition, where they rapidly harden. A good amalgam is as durable as gold, and resists equally well the attrition of mastication. It is of course far less costly. The great drawback of amalgam is that one that will retain its colour in all mouths has yet to be discovered, and even a slight discolouration is objectionable in front teeth. For front teeth the so-called osteo plastic stoppings are employed to a large extent, and consist of a powder and liquid which, combined, make a white paste which sets hard in a few minutes and retains its colour in the mouth. These stoppings are sufficiently hard to resist the wear of mastication, but the saliva has a slightly solvent action upon them and they require renewing every two or three years. Gutta percha stoppings are chiefly used for temporary stopping, etc., but is fairly durable in some cases, as in small cavities near the gum margin, etc.

Gutta percha, as used in dentistry, is prepared by the addition of a hydraulic cement which causes it to set hard in the mouth and is quite distinct from the so-called white enamel sold at the drug stores. This "white enamel," which is only ordinary white gutta percha, becomes indescribably offensive in the mouth and pollutes the breath terribly and, if introduced in a cavity

between the teeth, frequently by its expansive
power forces the teeth apart, causing them to
assume most unsightly positions, and possibly
their loss by driving the gums back from the
roots.

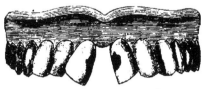

Fɪɢ. 47.—Showing two central teeth driven apart and the
rest of the teeth displaced by amateur stopping with ordinary
white gutta percha.

What are known as mineral or porcelain
inlays also make very artistic stoppings. The
lost portion of the natural tooth is replaced by
a small section of mineral tooth accurately
fitted and cemented in the cavity.

The mineral inlay is natural looking, and the
least easily detected of all stoppings, and is
especially suitable for small cavities in front
teeth.

Patients are of course not ordinarily qualified to judge of the relative merits of the various
materials and methods, nor of their special
applicability in individual cases, and cannot do
otherwise than to select a qualified dentist, and
submit to his judgment—very certain to be
better than their own—and, having done so, to
give him all the help in their power to secure

the good results desired by both. Good operations of any and all classes fail often because of a want of cleanliness on the part of the patient.

If the teeth decay because of unhealthy conditions of the mouth, produced either by constitutional or other causes, a continuance of

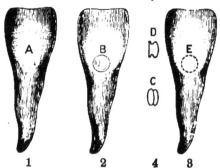

FIG. 48.—Porcelain Inlays.

1, Central tooth with small decayed cavity in the front (A).
2, Central tooth with cavity (B) prepared to receive porcelain inlay.
8, Central tooth with porcelain inlay (E) in position.
4, Prepared porcelain inlay, front of (C); transverse section of (D).

the same influences will produce further decay after the most thorough and most conservative local treatment. A tooth that has been filled or filed is not, therefore, to be supposed invulnerable to the attacks of destructive agents, and the dentist should not be held responsible for the patient's neglect. As a sick man requires more care than a healthy one, so a damaged tooth, even though repaired, needs more attention than a sound one.

Tartar or Salivary Calculus.

TARTAR consists of the earthy salts of the saliva which are deposited about the sides and the necks of the teeth. It first forms a light, soft, creamy layer which hardens and thickens until, in extreme cases, the teeth are almost entirely enveloped in it. It generally presents a dirty, yellow, bone-like appearance, but may

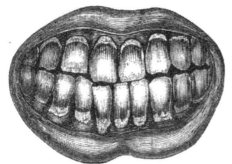

FIG. 49.—Showing a Mouth with accumulation of yellowish coloured Tartar collected about the necks of the teeth.

assume a brown, green, or black colour. It varies from an almost flinty hardness to a soft, friable consistency. As a rule its hardness is in inverse proportion to its quantity; with small deposits which have been collecting for a considerable time the tartar is usually dark and hard, while with large and rapidly growing deposits the tartar is light coloured and soft.

The hard tartar adheres to the teeth with

G

great tenacity, while the soft variety is easily removed. In fact it shows a tendency to break away spontaneously, leaving rough edges which excoriate the tongue and cheeks.

In young people the permanent teeth soon after their appearance through the gum may become disfigured by the deposition of dark

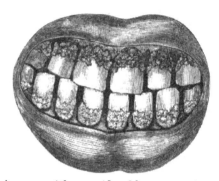

FIG. 50.—A case with considerable accumulation of rough dark yellow Tartar.

green pigment upon the surface of the enamel. The habitual use of the tooth-brush and the act of mastication gradually rub off the pigment and the teeth are restored to their proper colour. If, however, the disfigurement remains after the teeth are fully developed and the enamel has acquired density, the unsightly appearance may be removed by the dentist.

It is frequently found that the enamel is roughened and chalky looking under this deposit. If this is the case it may be smoothed and polished. This discolouration is possibly of vegetable origin, and is quite distinct from tartar.

The deposition of tartar does little or no injury to the enamel of the tooth, and is certainly not an exciting cause of decay in the teeth, but it is directly injurious to the gums, sockets, breath, secretions of the mouth, and to the general health. The first deposit irritates the gums; they inflame, perhaps suppurate, and recede; here they would stop and heal if it were not for the continued addition of tartar,

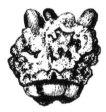

Fig. 51.—An Upper Molar lost through the accumulation of Tartar encroaching on the sockets.

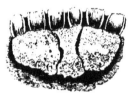

Fig. 52.—Six Front Teeth nearly covered with Tartar, and lost through its destructive effects on the alveoli (sockets).

which causes the gums to recede more and more. This deposition also encroaches upon the vessels affording vitality to the alveolar processes and the roots of the teeth; the devitalized processes are gradually absorbed, and finally, when they and the gums are both gone, the teeth become loose and fall out. So intolerably offensive does the breath become from some kinds of porous tartar which give lodgment to decomposing mucous and food, that it is almost insufferable.

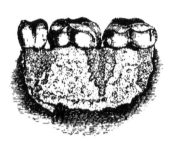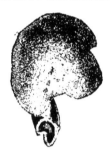

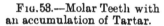

Fig. 53.—Molar Teeth with an accumulation of Tartar.

Fig. 54.—A collection of Tartar gathered on the root of an Upper Bicuspid.

The fluids of the mouth become vitiated, are taken into the stomach, which rebels at such a condiment; the blood becomes full of impurities, the system suffers, and often the best efforts of the physician fail while the cause exists.

An eminent writer, in his work on Dental Surgery, further enumerates the effects of tartar as follows: " Tumours and spongy excrescences of the gums of various kinds; necrosis and exfoliation of the alveolar processes, and of portions of the maxillary bones; hemorrhage of the gums; loss of appetite; derangement of the whole digestive apparatus; foul breath; catarrh; cough; diarrhea; diseases of various kinds in the maxillary antra and nose; pain in the ear; headache; melancholy, etc.

Add to these closure of the salivary ducts, periodontitis, alveolar abscess, and various sympathetic pains : think a little—and then resolve to
keep the teeth clean. There is one great means
of cure, and that is the operation of scaling
performed by the dentist."

The removal of the tartar or scaling, as the
operation is called, from the teeth is a painless
operation, and if skilfully performed cannot
possibly injure the teeth, and when we consider
the benefits derived from having the teeth clean
and the breath free from fetid taint, it is difficult to see how any one paying any regard to
their own welfare or the feelings of others can
for one moment object to it.

Extraction.

THE advance of knowledge in dental surgery,
the improvements in the treatment of decayed
teeth, the use of antiseptics in the nerve canals,
and recent improvements in crowning, render
it possible to save many teeth that would otherwise be doomed to extraction. Almost any
tooth can by persistent treatment be retained
and rendered useful for a time unless it is
absolutely loose; but in the case of badly
abscessed teeth the course of treatment required is protracted, and unfortunately occupies

more time than a busy patient can afford. While with nervous and delicate patients the strain of long operations is so exhausting that extraction becomes the only available remedy, especially when the risk is considered that after repeated antiseptic dressings, etc., spread over several weeks, there is still the possibility of failure to save the tooth and reduce the inflamed and abscessed socket to a reasonably healthy condition. When the extraction of a tooth is really necessary it is a folly to allow it to remain, causing pain and sleeplessness, preventing mastication and injuring the bodily health. The pain of extraction is not so great but what it can be faced by any ordinary individual with the exercise of a little courage, and even this pain can be avoided by the use of anesthetics.

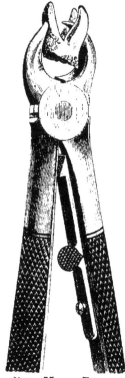

FIG. 55. — Forceps designed to extract stumps of upper molars when broken down to the level of the gum.

It is necessary that the forceps used should fit the teeth to be extracted, and as the teeth

differ greatly in shape a large number of instruments is required to meet the exigencies of
an ordinary practice, and not only is a special
instrument necessary for each tooth, but additional ones to extract teeth of varying size, or
whose form or position deviate from the normal.

Many consider the operation of extracting
teeth to be one that requires little skill, and are
willing to entrust their mouth for this purpose
to the tender mercies of the chemist's assistant
or any other individual who chooses to display
the legend, "Teeth Extracted," in his window;
but to become a really good operator in this
respect it is necessary not only to have had
considerable practice, but also to have . a
thorough anatomical knowledge of the teeth
and jaws, and of such deviations from their
normal condition as are likely to be met with
in practice.

Painless Extraction of the Teeth by Nitrous Oxide Gas.

NITROUS oxide, or laughing gas, was the
earliest discovered anesthetic, for as long ago
as 1799 Sir Humphry Davy made use of the
following words : " As nitrous oxide in its
extensive use seems capable of destroying
physical pain, it may probably be used with
advantage in operations where no great effusion

of blood takes place." This noteworthy observation produced no result, and the grand
idea that the peculiar properties of the gas
might be employed for the good of suffering
humanity lay fallow until the year 1844. In
that year at a scientific lecture delivered in
Connecticut, a local dentist noticed that a
gentleman under the influence of nitrous oxide
struck himself without experiencing any pain
from the blow. Next day he visited the lecturer in company with another dentist, and
asked that he might be placed under the gas.
Under its influence his fellow dentist pulled
out one of his firmest teeth without his feeling
it. Having experienced the result in his own
person this man, whose name was Wells,
speedily learned how to produce the gas, and
applied it with every success in a number of
dental cases. Unhappily he had not the
necessary courage and hardihood to resist the
opposition of the medical faculty. Offering to
perform a public operation with the gas, he did
so at a hospital in the presence of a large
number of sceptical and sneering doctors. For
some reason or other the patient cried out;
Wells was unnerved, the doctors laughed him
to scorn, and so great seems to have been his
mortification that he died shortly afterwards.

The lecturer however, Dr. Colton, would not

abandon his faith in the "laughing gas" so easily, after having once had his eyes opened by the unlucky Wells; and for twenty years he continued to urge its use upon the dentists in America. For long years, possibly fearing the fate of Wells, they all refused to have anything to do with it. At last he was successful, and having won the day in the United States, Dr. Colton visited Paris with a clean record of 20,000 cases without a single accident. The French faculty gave him but slight encouragement, but his cause was warmly espoused by Dr. Evans, who subsequently brought his apparatus to London, and administered the gas before the staff of the Dental Hospital.

Nitrous oxide is the safest, pleasantest, and simplest of all anesthetics hitherto discovered. Since its introduction in this country it has been used in millions of cases with unvarying success and immunity from accident. These virtues single it out from all other agents employed for the suppression of pain in dental operations, while the rapidity with which the patient recovers consciousness, and the absence of the disagreeable after-effects which follow the inhalation of chloroform, etc., are strong evidence of the entire absence of danger in the use of gas.

The administration of nitrous oxide gas is not

unpleasant to the patient; it is practically inodorous, but has a slightly sweet taste. No feeling of suffocation is felt while breathing it. The time occupied in obtaining a complete state of insensibility is about two minutes, and the duration of the insensibility is about thirty seconds to one minute. The patient rapidly recovers when the administration of the gas is stopped, and as a rule feels none the worse for the experience.

Considerable improvements have recently been made in the apparatus for the administration of gas, and modifications have been introduced for continuing its administration through the nose while the operation on the mouth is in progress, thus considerably lengthening the period of insensibility available, while a similar result is obtained by the administration of a mixture of nitrous oxide gas and oxygen, with the additional advantage that the resulting anesthesia is much quieter.

Patients frequently suffer from toothache for several days, losing their rest night after night, and at times even abstaining from food owing to the increased pain caused by eating. Finally in a fit of desperation, they visit a dentist and have the tooth extracted under gas; naturally they have fallen into a state of thorough physical and mental exhaustion. Upon recovery they usually attribute their collapsed state to the after-effects of the gas, not recognizing that whether they had taken gas or not they would have felt equally ill through the suffering they had undergone before the aching tooth was removed.

Women, when pregnant, will often suffer considerable pain from a decayed tooth under the delusion that their condition prohibits them having the tooth extracted, and this opinion is frequently shared by their medical attendant, but all dental authorities agree that pregnancy is no bar to the extraction of teeth, if necessary to relieve pain, especially under nitrous oxide gas. This anesthetic has been frequently used even when the confinement was imminent, and the tooth removed without injury either to the mother or child.

Use of Local Anesthetics in Dentistry.

UNDER nitrous oxide, chloroform and ether, the anesthesia is general, that is, the patient loses consciousness; but in the minor surgical operations only a small part requires to be deprived of sensation. From the very nature of it general anesthesia has more or less the elements of danger, from which local anesthesia is free. Many attempts have been made to discover a reliable local anesthetic, effectively annulling the pain of extraction without rendering the patient insensible. Electricity, ether spray, calorific fluid, and chloride of ethyl have been tried, and for one reason or another have proved failures in actual practice. Eucaine and cocaine are the only reliable local anesthetics in dentistry, and by the aid of these agents the operation of extracting teeth can be performed without pain and without loss of consciousness.

Cocaine.

COCAINE is the active principle of a plant *Erythroxylon Coca*, a native of Peru, the leaves of which were found to be in use by the Peruvians when that country was conquered by the Spaniards nearly four centuries ago. The natives ascribed to this plant the property of making them insensible to hunger, of adding to their strength and vigour, and of relieving oppressive respiration during mountain ascents. Specimens of the leaves were at various times sent to Europe, but the alkaloid was not obtained from them till 1860. The discovery was made by Neimann in the Vienna laboratory, and it was noted at that time that it had the property of rendering the tongue temporarily insensible at the point of contact, but beyond this its power of producing local anesthesia was un-

known till 1884, when Dr. Köller, of the Vienna
General Hospital, discovered its virtue in this
respect. Since that date its use as a local
anesthetic has spread with great rapidity, particularly for operations on the eye, for which
purpose cocaine has absolutely superseded all
other agents for the abolition of pain, as the delicate surface of that organ leads to the immediate
absorption of the drug. As regards the use of
cocaine in dentistry, the external application
of cocaine to the gum around the tooth makes
the surface of that membrane, after the lapse
of a few minutes, quite insensible to pricking
or scratching, and it is frequently thus applied
on wool with a view to the mitigation of the
pain of extraction; but its effect is then too
superficial: it is in fact only skin deep. To be
effectual the drug requires to be applied hypo-
dermically, i.e. injected beneath the skin.
When so used, there is first a feeling of
warmth, then insensibility of the part in the
neighbourhood of which the injection has
taken place, permitting the painless extraction
of the tooth. After the lapse of half an hour
the normal sensibility returns. Cocaine is thus
specially useful for the removal of broken-down
roots and other prolonged operations, for which
gas is unsuitable, owing to the short duration
of the insensibility it produces. Cocaine has

also been used in dentistry to deaden the
sensitiveness of exposed nerves in preparing
cavities of teeth previous to filling and, added
to the devitalizing agent used in the destruction
of the nerve in a decayed tooth, renders this
operation perfectly painless.

The quantity of cocaine used in the extraction of a tooth is very small. In *large* quantities
cocaine may be poisonous, and several alarmist
articles have appeared in the daily press, in-
spired by injury caused by the use of this drug
in conjunction with morphia, chloral, etc., by
habitual drug takers, many of whom consume
daily quantities far in excess of any amount
that could possibly be used for the legitimate
purposes of dental or general surgery.

A few practitioners have an unreasonable
prejudice against the use of cocaine owing
probably to the fact that when it was first
obtainable in this country, some fifteen years
ago, the cocaine commercially supplied was
a crude and impure pharmaceutical product
which, when dissolved, produced a turbid
solution in which small fragments of coca
leaves and stalks, particles of wood, grit, etc.,
were quite visible. The proportion of hygrin
and other soluble impurities was large. This
crude cocaine often in stale solutions was extensively, not to say recklessly, employed in far

larger doses than would be used to-day, under conditions that any one practically acquainted with the properties of cocaine would have known to have been unfavourable to its employment.

A number of cases in which alarming symptoms appeared were naturally met with, and led to the abandonment of the use of the agent altogether by some practitioners; but those who persevered in the use of the drug soon learnt that the so-called toxic effects of cocaine were the result of decomposed solutions and of impure cocaine, and could be avoided by the use of the pure drug freshly dissolved in sterilized water.

To-day cocaine is the most extensively employed anesthetic in the surgical treatment of the nose, throat, mouth and eyes, and was the agent employed in the eye troubles of her late Majesty Queen Victoria, and also in the operation for cataract performed on the late Rt. Hon. W. E. Gladstone. Its employment in such cases quite shows that it is a perfectly safe anesthetic in skilled hands; and this is confirmed by the authors' experience, which extends over 100,000 administrations for the extraction of teeth, etc., in the last fourteen years.

Eucaine.

EUCAINE is very similar in its properties to cocaine. It is a product of the chemical laboratory and is one of those complex chemical bodies for which we are indebted to the German chemical research. It was discovered in the course of experiments to make an artificial cocaine. Although a useful anesthetic it is practically innocuous even in large quantities; it can be used in cases where for any reason cocaine is objected to. It is injected into the gum in a manner similar to cocaine, and in a few moments renders the gum quite insensible, permitting the painless removal of the tooth. The authors have used eucaine in a large number of cases with very satisfactory results. It is slightly slower and less reliable in its action than cocaine, to which it is preferred by many authorities, and like cocaine is extensively used in dental and ophthalmic surgery.

Ether Spray and Ethyl Chloride.

ETHER spray was originally introduced by Sir B. W. Richardson, and has been used for many years as an obtundent in the extraction of the teeth. Pure sulphuric ether is thrown on the gum, at the sides of the tooth or teeth to be extracted, by a spraying apparatus worked by a small foot bellows. The intense cold produced rapidly freezes the gum and minimizes the pain of the operation. The greatest drawback to its employment in dentistry is the fact that the first shock caused by the cold spray being

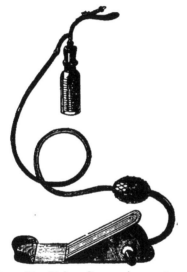

Fig. 56.—Ether Spray Apparatus.

thrown in the sensitive tooth is often nearly as painful as the actual extraction. Ether spray is now superseded by chloride of ethyl, which has precisely the same action as ether spray and is more effective and less unpleasant to the patient. For large and firm teeth it is of little use, but where a number of loose teeth

H

have to be extracted it proves a very useful
local anesthetic. It is generally supplied in
small glass bulbs having a minute opening at
the top through which, when held in the warm
hand the ethyl chloride is projected in a small
stream which is directed on the gum in the
neighbourhood of the tooth to be extracted.
The gum becomes blanched and anesthetized,
and the poignancy of the pain of extraction
considerably reduced.

Difficulties and Complications in the Extraction of Teeth.

LIKE other surgical operations the extraction
of teeth is at times attended with certain
difficulties and complications and the healing
of the gums may not proceed as favourably as
can be desired. Considerable resistance to
efforts to effect the removal of a tooth will
sometimes occur. This is naturally, though
not always, most frequently met with in those
of strong physique. Isolated teeth remaining
long after their neighbours are lost are always
more difficult to extract than those in series, as
the bone in the vacant sockets becomes consolidated around them.

Colyer (Lecturer on Dental Surgery to

the Charing Cross Hospital) says :—" It may perhaps be found impossible to remove the tooth. When this is the case it is better to dismiss the patient and to make a fresh attempt two or three days later. The tooth will probably be loose as a result of the inflammation and can be easily removed." [1]

The chief causes of undue resistance to efforts

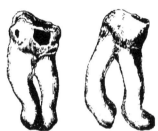

Fig. 57.—Lower Molar Teeth with roots enlarged by Exostosis.

of extraction are abnormal density of the bone, divergent or twisted roots, or the enlargement of the roots of the tooth brought about by a disease known as exostosis, which is met with very frequently where a gouty tendency exists. Broken-down teeth and roots are obviously the most difficult to extract, but with a good set of modern instruments, skilfully employed, the dentist's power to remove even the most unpromising-looking roots is surprising; but at the same time the occasional

[1] *Extraction of the Teeth.* Colyer.

fracture of a tooth and the inability to remove the roots at the same sitting are not proofs of want of skill.

Coleman (Examiner in Dental Surgery) says:—" A tooth, the attachments of which are of greater strength than its own cohesive force, must of necessity yield in the latter, as will a rotten carrot when attempted to be pulled from the ground. In such cases, should the remaining portion prove very firm, we may have to employ judgment as to the length of time for which we are to persevere in our efforts to remove it; it might turn out that we are attempting an impossibility, as evidenced at times by the abnormal form of its roots or growths upon them.

" It is extremely unpleasant to send a patient away with an aching tooth *in situ*, but in most cases we have found a temporary cessation of pain in a tooth, the removal of which has been attempted, whilst we may almost for certain give the assurance that, should the tooth again become tender it will also become somewhat loose."[1]

Fracture of the jaw has been known as a result of the extraction of a tooth, but with ordinary care in performing the operation such

[1] *Dental Surgery and Pathology.*

an occurrence is almost impossible except in cases where some extraordinary malformation of the jaw exists; but it is probable that the alveoli or thin bone surrounding the teeth is more or less injured in almost every case of extraction, and frequently small pieces come away adhering to the root of the tooth. This is of little importance, as the whole of this bone

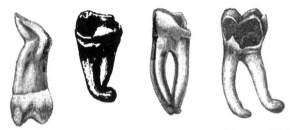

Fɪɢ. 58.—Teeth with curved roots which would cause difficulty in extraction.

is absorbed as the gums fall away subsequent to the extraction. Small detached portions of the socket should be removed after the tooth, but are likely to escape observation during the bleeding. These, if allowed to remain, may cause some slight irritation, but are sloughed off in the course of a few days as the socket heals. In the past, when the instrument known as the key was used in extracting teeth, it was not unusual for extensive fractures of the alveoli to occur, involving the sockets of perhaps two or three teeth in addition to the one it was intended to extract; but with the modern forceps the risk of alveolar injury is reduced to a minimum, and when it does occur is so slight that it may be disregarded, excepting so far as the removal of detached fragments are concerned.

Excessive Bleeding after Extraction.

PROLONGED and troublesome bleeding after the extraction of a tooth is by no means rare and is not necessarily dependent on the extent or nature of the wound. Bleeding is as likely to occur after a simple extraction as it is after the removal of a large and broken-down tooth, where considerable laceration of the gums has proved unavoidable. It is more frequently met with in cases where one tooth has been removed than it is after the more extensive operations undertaken to clear the mouth of teeth and fangs for the reception of artificial teeth. That a clean-cut wound with smooth edges bleeds more than a lacerated one is shown by the fact that a small cut inflicted by a razor or sharp knife bleeds profusely, while a torn wound of equal size from a jagged nail will hardly bleed at all. The skill or want of skill with which the operation of extraction has been performed has little influence on the amount of bleeding that follows. The result even of a small wound would be that the whole of the blood would be drained from the body were it not for the tendency of the blood vessels to contract and thus prevent its escape. The blood itself also has the property of becoming thick (coagulating). These two causes combined check the flow of the blood from the wound. Where the blood does not stop in reasonable time it is principally because from some cause the blood vessels fail to contract, for frequently in hemorrhage cases the blood will form a firm clot in the mouth, although the socket itself is filled with fluid blood. This want of the power of contraction in the smaller blood vessels is frequently a personal peculiarity and constitutes what is known as the "hemorrhagic diathesis." It is advisable where this tendency is known to exist to avoid as far as possible extracting the teeth and other operations leading to the effusion of blood.

Troublesome bleeding after the extraction of a tooth usually takes the form of secondary hemorrhage; that is, after the operation the bleeding ceases and the patient returns home. At the expiration of some hours the bleeding recommences. Generally the patient wakes up in the night and finds his pillow saturated with blood which continues to issue in a steady stream from the socket. The best course to adopt is to return to the dentist who extracted the tooth, and as a temporary expedient the blood can almost always be checked by soaking cotton wool in water and rolling it in a ball about the size of a large walnut, and placing this over the affected socket in such a manner that the wool is firmly held in position by the teeth of the opposite jaw when the mouth is closed. Of course if the opposing teeth are lost a larger piece of wool is required, so that the jaw itself produces a steady pressure on the socket. A bandage passed under the chin and over the head sufficiently tight to prevent the mouth being opened is preferable to trusting to the volition of the patient. It is advisable to pack a piece of dry wool in the socket itself before placing the wet ball of wool in its place. It is undesirable to give spirits or other stimulants to patients suffering from bleeding unless absolute collapse is threatened, as a slight feeling of faintness is often a prelude to the cessation of the hemorrhage; and stimulants, by reducing the arterial tension, increase the flow of blood. Professional assistance should be obtained at the earliest possible moment unless, of course, this palliative treatment results in the stoppage of the bleeding, and even then a return to the dentist who extracted the tooth, for his advice, is desirable.

Pain after Extraction.

AFTER the tooth has been extracted considerable pain may be experienced more or less constantly for several days. Coleman says :—

"We must bear in mind that pain set up by a diseased tooth does not always cease with its removal, and this is especially the case where inflammation has set up in, or extended to, its periosteum " (socket lining).

" The pain after the laceration of membranes in such a condition is, we can well comprehend, usually very acute and may last for several hours, according to the stage of inflammation at which the tooth was removed." [1]

In badly abscessed cases the discharge may continue from the sockets for some days and the gum surrounding it looks swollen, unhealthy and inflamed, the socket itself being occupied by a yellow slough and the breath rendered unpleasant by the discharge. Fomenting the mouth with hot solution of carbolic acid (20 to 30 drops of liquid carbolic acid to a tumbler of hot water) has proved the most satisfactory

[1] *Dental Surgery and Pathology.*

treatment in the authors' practice. This fomentation should be persevered with from 10 to 15 minutes at a time and repeated several times daily until the wound heals.

After a tooth has been extracted the bone of the socket can commonly be felt, and much pain and inflammation is often caused by the patient probing the empty socket with a penknife, pins and similar sharp instruments, frequently in an uncleanly condition; or by sticking the tongue or finger into the wound, under the delusion that there is a piece of the tooth left in. The thickness of the gum covering the bone is only about equal to that of a piece of wet wash leather, and as the socket comes up to the necks of the teeth the bone composing it can be both seen and felt in the cavity from which a large tooth like a molar has been extracted.

Where the fixing of the jaws (known as trismus) exists it is generally very important to remove the tooth causing it immediately, as there is a great probability of the abscess discharging through the cheek or under the chin and causing an unsightly and permanent disfigurement.

It is generally possible, by a little manipulating, to introduce the forceps; while, under the influence of nitrous oxide gas, the mouth can be opened by a " Mason's gag " and the tooth removed without difficulty. The face in these cases should not be poulticed, nor is it desirable to wait till the swelling subsides. Where the trismus is severe and the inflammation runs high, especially if the temperature of the patient is raised, every hour the tooth causing the trouble is allowed to remain increases the danger of the abscess opening externally and causing permanent disfigurement. Directly the tooth is extracted the pus is discharged through the empty socket and the patient regains his normal temperature in a few hours.

Necrosis.

NECROSIS, or death of a portion of the jaw bone, may occur after the extraction of a tooth, especially in cases where severe inflammation and abscess have existed. The disease may be confined to the socket of the tooth extracted or involve a considerable portion of the jaw bone. Sir John Tomes says :—

"Necrosis of a portion of the bone may follow upon the extraction of a tooth, however skilfully this has been performed; and it must not be supposed that the operator is to blame for the advent of necrosis after the extraction of a tooth.

" The conditions leading to necrosis are, in

the great majority of cases, developed previously to the removal of the tooth, and are
quite independent of its removal; the necrosis
would generally have been quite as sure, and
perhaps even more extensive, had the tooth
been left in. There is not the smallest reason
for believing that the removal of a tooth should
be deferred because the tissues around it are in
a state of acute inflammation or suppuration.
If the tooth be the exciting cause of the mischief, there is no excuse for delaying its extraction for a single moment; and the opinion
to the contrary, held though it be by a number
of medical men, is in no degree shared by
dentists; and, being based on no evidence
whatever, must take rank in the category of
popular errors." [1]

The indications that attend necrosis are
toothache and tenderness in one or more teeth,
swelling of the face. The gum becomes thickened
over the diseased part, and of a deep red colour;
pus oozes out between the edge of the gum and
the teeth. After a time the gum separates
from the bone, which then becomes exposed.
The discharge becomes very profuse and very
offensive. After a time, generally a few weeks,
the dead bone separates from the living and is
thrown off (exfoliated), and recovery takes place.

[1] *System of Dental Surgery.*

Premature Loosening and Falling out of the Teeth.

WITH those whose dental organs have success-fully resisted the ravages of decay a gradual wasting of the bony sockets, accompanied by a corresponding recession of the gum, keeps pace with those general changes which attend the advance towards old age. The necks of the teeth become exposed and the gum ridges sink lower and lower till the whole of the roots are uncovered and the teeth fall out.

The ridges of the jaw waste till in some instances the upper jaw becomes nearly flat, and the lower is reduced to a mere bar of bone almost flat topped. This absorption of the alveoli, as it is called, is unfortunately not only met with in advanced age. It is occasion-ally met with in early middle life, and antidates by a long period any other sign of approaching senility. It is difficult to account in some cases for this premature recession of the gum, as the inflammation of the gums and tartar are both absent, and it is frequently found that teeth which have no antagonists in the mouth through their opposing teeth in the opposite jaw having been lost, are more liable to loosen than those in full use, and the

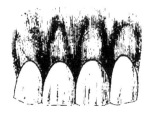

FIG. 59.

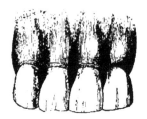

FIG. 60.

Fig. 59 shows the gum in its normal state passing up in points between the teeth.

Fig. 60 shows the teeth and gum in an early stage of pyorrhea alveolaris; the delicate festooning of the gum round and between the necks of the teeth has been lost.

molars and bicuspids will often thus be shed while the front teeth remain perfectly firm. When the premature loosening of the teeth has occurred it is more usual to find that it is the result of a disease of a more active and inflammatory nature known as pyorrhea alveolaris.

One of the earliest symptoms of this disease is a thickening and rounding of the edge of the gum, which ceases to adhere to the neck of the tooth.

As the disease progresses the tooth becomes

detached from the soft parts to a considerable
depth, forming a kind of sulcus or pocket containing a small quantity of pus.

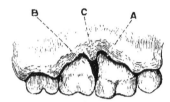

Fig. 61.—The receding gum, showing an early stage of pyorrhœa
alveolaris; the pocket exists at A C B.

A ring of dirty green tartar generally sur-
rounds the neck of the tooth. At the bottom
of this sulcus an extremely minute exposure of
the edge of the alveolus exists. This free

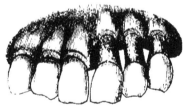

Fig. 62.—A case where the gums and sockets of three front teeth
are badly affected by pyorrhea alveolaris, while the corresponding
teeth on the opposite side remain comparatively healthy.

edge of bone is continually wasting away,
and thus the socket is ultimately disintegrated
and the tooth lost. This exposure of the bone
is shown in fig. 64 slightly exaggerated for the
purpose of illustration; the edge of bone
exposed is really microscopic in its proportions.

The breath is frequently rendered very offensive, and neuralgic pains are often experienced. The gums are inflamed and bleed readily. This disease, formerly known as " scurvy of the gums," often arises in otherwise healthy

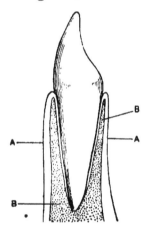

FIG. 63.

Section showing tooth and gum in healthy state.

a, The gum.
b, The bony walls of the socket.

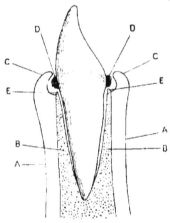

FIG. 64.

Section showing tooth and gum affected by pyorrhea alveolaris.

a, The gum.
b, The bony walls of socket exposed at E.
c, The rounded and inflamed edge of the gum.
d, The sulcus with a small deposit of tartar.

people who have hardly passed the period of middle life, and whose teeth have been exceptionally free from decay.

The treatment of pyorrhea alveolaris is to a great extent palliative and directed to the alleviation of the more distressing symptoms rather than the cure of the disease. Thus astringent mouth washes such as tannin and chlorate of potash will reduce the sponginess and congestion of the gums, while the use of carbolic acid (one drachm to one pint of water) or of listerine or other disinfectants, will do much to remove the unpleasantness from the breath. The progress of the disease can be checked by treating the gum round the necks of the teeth with iodine, aromatic sulphuric acid, cupric sulphate, and other agents; but these powerful escharotics can only be used by a dental surgeon. The removal of the tartar is a necessary preliminary, and the utmost cleanliness must be observed, the teeth being brushed frequently with a soft brush. A slight bleeding of the gums caused by cleaning, if not excessive, can be disregarded, as it probably is beneficial rather than otherwise in its effects, and tends to reduce the inflammation.

In an editorial article on pyorrhea alveolaris, *The British Journal of Dental Science,* January 15, 1902, says : " This disease is one of the most hopeless conditions of the mouth with which we are called upon to deal. At one time comparatively rare, it has of late years become appallingly common, and it seems to be extending its ravages to subjects in early adult life, to those whose vitality ought to be in its

highest vigour. Much has been written concerning its cause, course, and treatment, but as
regards the first and last named, we are still
much in the dark.

" Strict cleanliness, frequent visits to the
dentist for the removal of calculus, and brisk
brushing of the gums undoubtedly retard the
disease, but as far as our experience goes, any
relaxation of this discipline is attended by
fresh onslaughts of the disease.

" Fixation of the loosened teeth to each other,
to sound ones, or to an apparatus fixed in the
mouth, has often been tried, and with varying
success.   But is such treatment the best for
the health and welfare of the patient ?   The
chief function of the teeth is the masticatory
one.   How is this to be performed when a
number of loose and tender teeth are joined
together in this way ?

" If the teeth have arrived at such a state
the remedy is extraction, followed by a clean
healthy gum and a clean healthy palate.   Our
aim ought not to be to preserve the natural
teeth at any price, but to study the best interests
of our patients' health, and if the disease is so
far advanced as to be desperate, the offending teeth should be removed, and the mouth
rendered fit by artificial means to do the work
for which it is designed."

Erosion of the Teeth.

DENTAL erosion is a disease resulting in the wasting away first of the enamel and then of the dentine of the tooth, quite distinct from

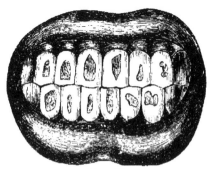

FIG. 65.

caries, as during the progress of the disease the affected spot presents a smooth, highly polished and sensitive surface. Erosion may

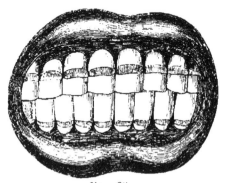

FIG. 66.

appear as irregular shaped excavations in the enamel of the teeth (fig. 65). Or it may pass in a broad band over several contiguous teeth, producing the appearance of the teeth having been filed away by a half round file and afterwards polished, fig. 66.

The causes of erosion are obscure; it is possibly in some cases the result of unsuitable tooth powders, and in others the acidity of the secretions of the mouth exercising a solvent action on the surface of the teeth.

Dental Hygiene.

IT is remarkable that among even well-to-do people the necessity for keeping the mouth and the teeth in a healthy condition is hardly recognized, and little cared for. Many times persons who are driven to consult their dentist on account of an aching tooth are horrified when they are told their teeth " are in a dreadful state," and resent it. They do not realize that of no portion of the human frame can it be said more truly than of the teeth that, " as you sow, so shall you reap." It is a hard matter to convince those in robust health that vitiated secretions, or habits of neglect and carelessness entail the decay of their teeth; while the crippled state of the teeth in its turn leads to a general enfeeblement of health. The rapid progress which microscopy and more especially bacteriology have made during the last few years has shown us that many diseases are communicated from one individual to another by means of extremely minute organisms, and further physiological chemistry has revealed to us that for such micro-organisms to exist, propagate and flourish, certain environments are requisite. In the mouth, with its constant condition of warmth and moisture, the micro-organisms are placed in the most favourable condition for development and multiplication, so that by the neglect of the ordinary laws of cleanliness, removal of particles of food about and between the teeth, and the omission to use frequently an antiseptic wash, the mouth becomes a mere breeding chamber for poisonous bacteria and micro-cocci. One often hears it said that "bad teeth run in families," and this belief, like all fatalistic doctrines, undoubtedly does harm by rendering persons callous, and so checking any inclination they might have possessed towards careful cleansing of the mouth.

But the truth of the matter is not accurately expressed by this formula, but rather by one which declares that an inherited bias towards early decay exists in families. In these families, if more strenuous efforts are employed and greater care taken in the daily ablutions of the mouth and teeth after every meal, the tendency to the early supervention of caries may be, and often is, over-ridden, and the teeth remain healthy for a long time. Were it possible to keep the teeth perfectly clean, decay would never occur, but owing to the form and contiguity of the teeth it is utterly impossible to cleanse them so thoroughly as to entirely dislodge the organisms that originate decay, but the nearer we can secure to the mouth an ideal state of cleanliness, the greater the chance we have of retaining our teeth in a healthy and useful condition.

That cleanliness is a prevention of decay is shown by the fact that teeth never decay on the cutting edges or surfaces that are sub- jected to the friction of the tongue and lips, unless some depression or fissure has previously existed.

Decay always originates between the teeth where they come in contact with or close to the gum, where, even with the greatest care, some small amount of food collects, or mucus can gather and decompose and form a nidus for the germs of decay to multiply and to attack the enamel of the tooth.

The means by which cleanliness can be secured to the mouth is by brushing with a

brush of suitable hardness not only the fronts,
but the backs of the teeth, and inside and across
the grinding surfaces of the molars, at least
twice a day, using some good tooth paste or
dentifrice once daily. The frequent passing of
a thread of floss silk between the teeth will
clear away many particles that the brush
cannot reach, while a mouth-wash and gargle of
listerine is both agreeable and beneficial for its
antiseptic properties. Simply brushing the teeth
without using a dentifrice will not prevent them
becoming discoloured. A tooth powder for a
healthy mouth should be merely a mechanical
agent possessing a hardness sufficient for the
removal of slight accumulation of food, mucus,
etc., without liability to injure the enamel; it
should be slightly antiseptic and free from
acidity and from rough and gritty ingredients
such as powdered pumice-stone, charcoal, etc.
Most of the brushes in the market are too large
and too stiff. Those known as the "Pierrepont
thorough cleaning" are certainly the most effective tooth brushes that can be obtained. They
are sold in pairs—one brush for the inside and
another for the outside of the teeth.

Much harm is frequently done to teeth by too
vigorous brushing with dentifrices containing
pumice powder, and cases are occasionally met
with in practice where the enamel is worn quite

through, and the dentine exposed. Care is necessary in brushing the teeth to cleanse them all over rather than in the expenditure of muscular force on the front of the mouth alone. The upper teeth should be brushed downward and the lower upward, as well as from side to side. The articulating faces of the teeth should be brushed with the same care as other

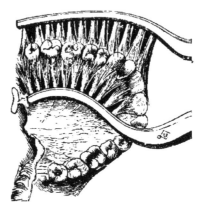

Fig. 67.

surfaces. The best time to use a dentifrice is before retiring at night.

During the waking hours the various movements of the tongue and muscles of the mouth in speech and otherwise, the constant salivary secretion and the mastication of food, all tend to prevent the chemical changes which during sleep take place without hindrance. Lime water [1] forms an excellent wash for weak teeth showing a tendency to decay, especially in young persons and where the saliva has an acid reaction. Teeth that become tender to the touch round the necks close to the gum are rendered less sensitive by the daily use of a

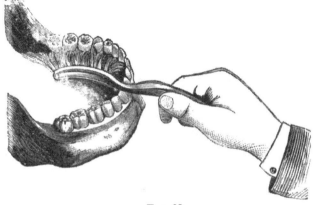

FIG. 68.

lime-water mouth wash. Its peculiar value consists in the fact that it is alkaline and neutralizes the effects of acids. Food may contain or become acid, or the saliva may be acid, a condition that frequently exists where the patient is debilitated.

Those who object to lime water because of

[1] Prepared by placing a piece of freshly burnt lime about the size of a hazel nut in a quart bottle of water, and shaking. It is then allowed to settle and the clear solution used. It must be kept tightly corked.

its unpleasant taste may remove this objectionable feature by using with it a few drops of eau de Cologne or rose water. A good mouth wash for spongy and bleeding gums is made by preparing a saturated solution of tannin in eau de Cologne, using about half a teaspoonful to a wine glass of hot water.

A teaspoonful of the tincture calendulae to a glass of water makes a pleasant mouth wash for use after the removal of tartar from the teeth.

Tincture of myrrh, so often prescribed, is merely a scent and is absolutely useless as a mouth wash.

Greater care of the teeth is necessary in sickness than in health, and irregular and crowded or weak teeth need much more attention to keep them in a wholesome state than those more regularly arranged and better organized.

Dental Dyspepsia.

" ALTHOUGH dentists are seldom consulted for trouble connected with the alimentary tract, they yet frequently have opportunities of seeing for themselves the harmful effects produced by neglect of the welfare of the teeth. The public in general, and the general run of the medical profession are scarcely alive to the part played by diseased teeth in producing indigestion. Where the teeth are imperfectly adapted for due mastication, from one cause or another, the owner of those teeth will infallibly suffer in his health. Children who are as careless of their teeth as their parents and nurses allow them to be—and that too often is careless to the verge of utter neglect—suffer not only in their childish persons, but even pass on to adolescence harmful habits formed in early childhood.

"It is far easier for a child to bolt his food, and say nothing about his toothache, than to face the supposed horrors of a visit to the dentist and all that that entails. The habit of bolting is soon acquired, and only broken after great trouble and self control. Nor are the evils more marked among children. Busy men, whose teeth are sound, often through carelessness and hurry scarcely use them at all; the food is bolted and the teeth soon suffer alike from an improper performance of function, and as a result of chronic congestion, which attacks the mucous membrane of the alimentary tract from the lips to the stomach and intestines. In cases where the teeth are tender mastication becomes neglected altogether or is very imperfectly performed, and done almost ex-

clusively on one side of the mouth. We no
longer seize or tear our food with our teeth,
but it is necessary for us to crush and grind it
by lateral and to and fro movements of the
jaws. Nor can the due amount of crushing or
grinding be carried out unless these actions of
the jaws are efficiently performed. The presence of fetid material in the mouth, whether
arising from necrosed stumps or carious teeth,
is a sure cause of dyspepsia. Dental dyspepsia
must be recognized and treated by the dentist.
Times out of number do patients get treated
by the medical advisers with bismuth or
alkalies or what not, when a few visits to a
dentist would have cured the disease. The
dentist is often asked to remove an aching
tooth. The most casual glance at the tongue
convinces him that not only is the aching
member at fault, but that also many of its
neighbours are also diseased. Under these
circumstances the dentist is quite justified in
promising a cure of the chronic dyspepsia if
the patient will submit to the removal of the
offending teeth, and their substitution by artificial ones which will be capable of making
mastication something more than an idle sham.
The public need educating in this respect,
and their eyes opened to the casual relation-
ship in which bad teeth, tender teeth, edentulous

jaws, and sore mouth, tongue or gums, have to dyspepsia." [1]

Artificial Teeth : Historical Sketch.

THE history of first efforts to replace the loss of natural teeth by artificial substitutes is lost in the remote past, for long before the Christian era records show that dentures constructed of human teeth or the teeth of the lower animals, secured in the mouth by gold wires, were in use among the Romans; and in a law promulgated B.C. 450, forbidding the burial of gold and jewels with the dead, exception is made in the case of gold wires serving to maintain the teeth. The museum of the town of Corneto, near Civita Vecchia, possesses two small dentures with artificial teeth, one of which was found near an Etrurian tomb dating back to four or five centuries before the Christian era; the other is from a Roman tomb of the same period. These pieces are carved out of the teeth of animals and fixed upon a ribbon of thin and very soft gold.

Nevertheless, we do not possess precise data relating to the practice of dentistry before Cornelius Celsus, who was born twenty-five or thirty years before our era at Rome, or at Verona, and died forty-five or fifty years after

[1] *British Journal of Dental Science.*

Christ, and from these early times until the eighteenth century probably no material advance was made in the construction and adaptation of artificial teeth.

Pierre Fauchard, in a work published in Paris in 1728, was the first to offer any satisfactory directions for the construction of plates to remedy fissure of the palate (cleft palate), and Bourdet, 1757, was amongst the earliest to construct and adapt whole sets of artificial teeth. These sets, composed of ivory and natural teeth, soon became useless. The ivory palate being acted upon by the fluids of the mouth became rough, dark-coloured, and offensive, while the natural teeth mounted upon it rotted away with great rapidity, necessitating the renewal of the denture every twelve or eighteen months. These undesirable qualities of ivory and natural teeth, foreign to the mouth, led to no practical attempt to the manufacture of artificial teeth from a mineral compound until the year 1774, when a French apothecary named Duchâteau conceived the idea and lost no time in putting it into execution. Taking a dentist named Dubois de Chemant into his confidence, they repaired to a French porcelain manufacturer, and here, conjointly, the earliest known attempt at the manufacture of mineral teeth was made.

The first efforts of Duchâteau and Dubois de Chemant terminated in failure, although the former received the thanks of the French Academy of Surgery for his laudable endeavours. While Duchâteau, presumably chilled by disappointment, seems to have abandoned the idea or considered it too remote to be worth persuing, Dubois de Chemant preserved it fresh in his mind, and in 1787 resumed his experiments in the hope of producing some substance impermeable to the secretions of the mouth. With official help he obtained the privilege of experimenting in the Government porcelain factory of Sevres. Experts in the art gave him the full benefit of their experience ; a small furnace was built for his use, and after patient investigation the material was evolved which was destined to play such an important part in the dentistry of the future.

The success of Dubois de Chemant provoked a storm of ill-favoured opposition. Leading French dentists of the day fancied they foresaw the enrichment of the inventor at the expense of their own practices. The news that an incorruptible artificial tooth had been discovered shook the orthodox practitioner with alarm. Duchâteau, too, who had disagreed with Dubois de Chemant, was chagrined at this unexpected success, and, joining the attack, brought a law-

suit against his former partner, claiming priority
of invention. Dubois de Chemant began to
experience that to be renowned is not always to
be happy, and that to labour for the improvement of human conditions is far from an un-
mixed blessing. His grateful *confrères* harassed
him with villainies, contrived to destroy his
furnace in the hope of wrecking any future
successes, and left nothing undone to secure his
downfall. Thanks to the good genius which
seems to have attended him throughout, the
designs of his enemies were foiled. The case
for Duchâteau broke down. M. Danet, the
Assayer at the French Mint, who all along took
a vital interest in the work of Dubois de
Chemant, was instrumental in obtaining a new
furnace, which Dubois de Chemant had constructed in his own house. The outbreak
of the French Revolution drove him from
France, and coming to England he established
himself in London some time during the closing
decade of the eighteenth century in Frith Street,
Soho.

Dubois de Chemant left behind him a book
which he called *A Dissertation on Artificial
Teeth*. De Chemant's teeth were not mounted
in gold or ivory plates, but both teeth and gums
were in one piece, and composed of the same
material, but their weight and brittleness were

obstacles to their general use, and we find later that they had fallen utterly into disrepute.

David Wemyss Jobson, Dentist in Ordinary to His Majesty King William IV., in his work on the teeth in 1834, says :—

" Artificial teeth have also of late years been made from porcelaneous substances and, under the name of ' mineral ' and ' terro-metallic ' teeth, have afforded an extensive range for empirical deception. The attraction held out is, they are alleged to be ' incorruptible,' by which term the unwary are entrapped and led to believe that teeth of this description are much more durable than the old ones (i.e. natural teeth artificially used).

" The very reverse is the case ; for although they are not subject to change of colour, yet they are in every instance so brittle as to be easily broken off on coming in contact with those of the opposite jaw. When these mineral or china teeth were first introduced, the most ex- travagant expectations were then formed from them, although few, or rather none, of the advantages they were supposed to possess have been realized, and they are now considered a complete failure. They have never been much used by the leading dentists of the day."

The condition under which a dental practice was conducted in 1830 is graphically described

K

by Mr. Daniel Corbett, Dental Surgeon, pre-
siding at the annual meeting of the British
Dental Association held in Dublin in 1888.
He stated : "Six weeks was the usual time
spent in the manufacture of a complete denture
when working bone and natural teeth. When
human teeth were in fashion, our supply
was usually had from the graveyard, and I
recollect what attention was paid to the grave-
digger at his periodical visits to my father's
residence with his gleanings from the coffins he
chanced to expose in the discharge of his avocation. His visits were generally at night, and
no hospitable duty in which my father might
chance to be engaged was permitted to interfere
with the reception of.this ever welcome visitor
into the *sanctum sanctorum* of the house."

The gravediggers every Monday morning
made their way to the dental depôts, each with
his sack on his back containing the ghastly
burdens collected during the previous week.

At this time of day we can scarcely realize
the horror of the scene of these men bringing
the jaws which they had turned up in "God's
acre" in their daily avocation; but mankind
required teeth, and to meet the need most of
those put in the mouth came from the jaws of
the dead.

It is said that the Battle of Waterloo furnished its quota of teeth ; but battles do not occur every day, and the bulk of the teeth that were used came from the graveyard and the hospital, and a lucrative trade it was !

Separate mineral teeth, designed to be mounted on gold or other plates, which finally gave the death blow to the use of the gleanings of the graveyard, were the invention of a M. Audibran, of Paris, and were introduced into this country by Mr. Corbett, senr., and their manufacture was taken up by Mr. Claudius Ash, of London, in 1837, who rapidly wrought a marvellous improvement in their strength and beauty, and severed once and for all the grave-diggers' connection with the dental surgery.

The introduction of gold plates for mounting artificial teeth early in the last century consti-tuted an important advance in the progress of prosthetic dentistry, but it had little effect on the cost. Artificial teeth still remained luxuries that only the very wealthy could afford, but the introduction of vulcanite and the general adop-tion of mineral teeth in the middle of the cen-tury wrought a veritable revolution in dentistry, by reducing the cost of production and placing artificial teeth of some description within the reach of all classes.

Prosthetic Dentistry.

THE replacement of the lost organs by artificial substitutes is one of the most important branches of the dentist's art, and many important points have to be kept in view. It is necessary that he should study carefully the requirements of each particularly, for there are no two cases alike, and a set of teeth that would be well adapted to the mouth of one person in point of utility, form and expression, would produce great imperfection and even distortion in the mouth of another. Hence the great importance of the most careful discrimination between the various requirements of different persons in this branch of dental practice.

The different functions of the natural teeth with reference to mastication, enunciation, articulation and restoration of the natural form and expression of the mouth and face should all be fully considered. From the taking of the impression, through all the different stages of the work to the final completion of a denture, various causes may occur which might prevent a successful result. Therefore, in order to avoid a failure from any of these causes, let us look for a moment at the acquirements necessary for one to possess who is to replace those organs which nature had previously formed; for whatever be the mode employed he will have to learn that it is the height of art to conceal art. This, together with practical utility, should be the great point to attain in the construction of artificial dentures. To reach these points requires the skill and perception of an artist, the manipulation and experience of an expert, together with thorough mental training and scientific research. Some new phase is encountered in each succeeding case as, for instance, in the length, size, form, position, and adaptation of the teeth, together with the lighter or darker shades and tones of the teeth and gums, all of which should be of a character suited to the age, complexion, and expression of the person for whom they are intended, thus producing one harmonious blending of all the features of the face of his patient. A broad and square or oval face, a large coarse featured man or a delicately organized woman, a miss of eighteen or a matron of fifty, a brunette or a blonde—these and other varieties present as many differing types, with teeth corresponding in size, shape, colour, and density. If, then, teeth correlated in their characteristics to those which nature assigns to one class be inserted in the mouth of one whose physical organization demands a different style, the effect cannot be otherwise than displeasing to the eye, whether the observer be skilled in perception or only intuitively recognizes inharmony without understanding the cause. It is quite possible in the adaptation of artificial teeth for the skilled dentist to avoid offending the eye trained to observe nature and to add to usefulness the charm of beauty.

The Adaptation of Artificial Teeth.

THE adaptation of artificial teeth is not painful nor is it necessary to submit to the removal of the teeth that remain in the mouth. The lost teeth can be restored without in any way interfering with those that remain intact. With reference to the extraction of the roots of decayed and broken-down teeth, whether their removal is necessary depends upon circumstances. Certainly where they are abscessed and continually emitting an offensive discharge their removal is to be desired for salutary reasons, entirely apart from the adaptation of artificial teeth; but in many cases healthy roots can be treated (as in crown and bridge work) and rendered useful as a support to the artificial denture.

The process of adaptation consists in taking an impression of the mouth in a soft plastic compound prepared for the purpose. From this a facsimile of the jaws is reproduced and the artificial teeth are prepared to suit the individual

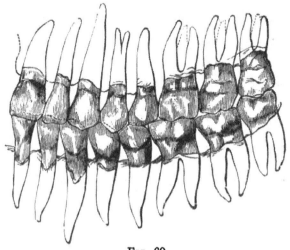

FIG. 69.

peculiarities of the case and have then to be inserted in the mouth. They are retained securely in their position by atmospheric pressure (suction) or other means, and can be removed and replaced by the patient without difficulty.

The time most favourable for the insertion of artificial teeth is as soon after the loss of the natural ones as the state of the mouth will permit before the facial expression has had time to alter, as the cheeks and lips are apt to become modified by the long absence of teeth, so that it is impossible to restore the original contour to the face. When the loss is partial the restoration of those teeth that have been lost is often the best means of preserving the rest, as a natural tooth left without an antagonist is apt to protrude from its socket and become loose, while the decay or the removal of the back teeth results in the destruction of the entire set. The cause of this can be seen in fig. 69, which represents the teeth closed in their natural position, the front upper teeth slightly overlapping the lower. The loss of the back teeth, by allowing the jaws to approach more closely, rapidly forces the upper teeth outward, causing them to become elongated and irregular, producing an unsightly protrusion of the mouth.

The lower teeth are forced inwards and also loosen and fall out. Figs. 70 and 71 show sectional views illustrating the result of the loss of the back teeth.

The teeth also act as conservators of the lungs, and organs of voice, preventing the breath, in the act of speaking, from being exhausted too rapidly. Those who have lost their teeth find continued speaking fatiguing, as each utterance empties the mouth of air, and more rapid breathing is necessary to keep up the supply. This induces a feeling of distress and is apt to produce a chronic cough, especially dangerous in those who suffer from weakness of the chest.

The disfigurement to the personal appear-

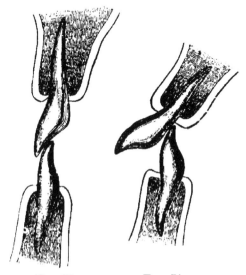

Fig. 70.   Fig. 71.

Fig. 70 shows the central incisors of the upper and lower jaws closing normally with the cutting edge of the upper tooth slightly overlapping the lower.

Fig. 71 shows the effect of the loss of the back teeth on the incisors. The whole force of mastication falling on the front teeth drives the upper outwards thus permitting the jaws to approach each other, until the lower tooth bites on the gum at the back of the upper.

ance, although the most obvious, is the least important injury inflicted by the loss of the teeth, and so fully is this recognized by the medical authorities of the present day that the restoration of the teeth to a serviceable condition by stopping the natural teeth where decayed, and by replacing by artificial teeth where lost, is regarded as indispensable in the treatment of digestive, lung and throat diseases.

The Construction of Artificial Teeth.

THERE are several bases used for the construction of artificial dentures—gold, silver, platinum, palladium silver, aluminium, vulcanite and celluloid. Which of these bases is best in a given case depends upon the nature and extent of the loss to be supplied, the age and physical characteristics of the patient, and the condition of the mouth. No one of these bases is always the best, and no authoritative opinion governing all cases can be therefore given, although for partial cases, especially for young persons, a gold denture can be confidently recommended. The advantages of gold are that plates can be made thinner and smaller than is the case with other bases. It is durable and can be re-modelled or repaired with the greatest facility, should the mouth undergo any alteration.

Gold is of course the most costly base, and thus is placed beyond the reach of many. Fortunately other less expensive plates are equal to gold in practical utility and durability. Dental alloy, known as dental platinum, is a base largely used in the construction of artificial teeth as a substitute for gold. It is composed of an alloy of platinum and silver, but owing to the largely increased price of pure platinum it is not now materially cheaper than gold. Palladium, formerly extensively used, but displaced by dental alloy, has lately been re-introduced; it is of a silvery grey colour and does not corrode in the mouth. Silver is unsuitable for the construction of artificial teeth, as it blackens and corrodes in the mouth, owing to its being acted upon by the sulphur existing in the saliva.

Attempts have been made to adapt aluminium to the mouth, but, owing to its softness and to the difficulty of soldering it, without practical success. It is used in conjunction with vulcanite, but it is very uncertain in its behaviour in the mouth, sometimes lasting without appreciable change for years, while in other cases it becomes corroded and roughened and wastes away with great rapidity. This wasting is probably the result of a slight contamination with antimony, which exists in much of the aluminium sold as "pure." The great recommendation possessed by aluminium is its lightness, but its softness prevents it displacing the more expensive metals in the dental laboratory.

There are some cases where the gums and
bone (consequent upon the loss of teeth, as in
fig. 73) have entirely receded. In such instances

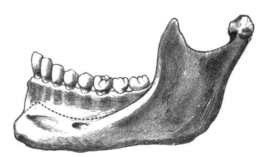

Fɪɢ. 72.

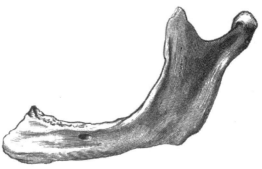

Fɪɢ. 73.

Fɪɢ. 72.—The lower jaw of an adult, with the teeth and sockets
in their normal state.   The dotted line shows the extent to
which the bone falls away after the loss of the teeth.
Fɪɢ. 73.—The same jaw after the teeth have been lost and the
sockets have fallen away, causing the recession of the gums.

gold would be insufficient, as a material resembling the gum is requisite, possessing such
qualifications of lightness and durability that it
can be recommended to restore the sunken

gums and return to the face the natural contour. This is best effected by the improved
form of vulcanite, now in use because it is
imperishable, and affords absolute resistance to
the action of the acids, and is consequently not
liable to corrode with the saliva. Its inherent
toughness, firmness, tenacity and fine texture

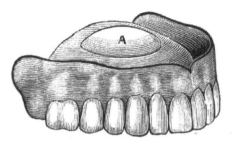

Fig. 74.—Vulcanite suction, upper set of teeth. A, vacuum
chamber.

make it peculiarly adapted for suction; it is
not likely to break, wear away, nor become
rough, and is susceptible of an elegant finish.
It forms one undivided piece of mechanism,
without seams or crevices for the lodgment of
secretion, thus securing purity to the mouth.
To reduce the vulcanite to a hard substance
when it has been moulded to the form required,
steam pressure is used, which converts it into a
perfectly compact substance as strong as metal.

It frequently occurs that after going on
without giving trouble for some years, the
natural teeth of an individual fail from one

cause or another and are lost in rapid succession, often at intervals of a few months, necessitating the addition of new teeth to the artificial denture and the ultimate renewal of the case is required at a much earlier date than it would have been had the mouth been in more stable condition.

Vulcanite is generally the best base to use under these circumstances, as it is more easily repaired and altered than any other material. It affords greater support to loose and shaky teeth, and it is less costly should it be imperative to replace it by a new case. Artificial dentures are also constructed of combinations of gold or platinum with vulcanite. The metal is frequently worked up in the palate to strengthen and stiffen the vulcanite plate. Thus used, the gold or platinum adds materially to the durability of the case, and enables the practitioner to make a thinner and slighter denture than could be otherwise trusted to. Another form of combination work is where the teeth are mounted on vulcanite attached to a gold or platinum plate. This form of work is rarely to be recommended, as it makes a very heavy case and more costly than vulcanite, and absolutely inferior in practical utility, while it is difficult to repair, because in the event of the metal plate requiring to be soldered the heat employed destroys the vulcanite to which the teeth are attached, and therefore necessitates remodelling the case should the slightest repair be required to the plate.

Although lightness is a usual *desideratum* in a denture it is not always so, as a small increase in the weight of a lower case occasionally affords

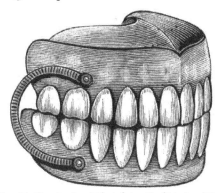

FIG. 75.—Full set of artificial teeth fitted with springs.

valuable aid in overcoming the resistance of the muscles of the cheeks and tongue, and in enabling the case to be retained with comfort without attachments to the remaining teeth, or the use of spiral springs, by the force of gravity alone. This extra weight may be obtained by inserting a core of metal in the centre of the vulcanite, or by constructing what is known as a " cast metal denture." These dentures are cast in one piece from an alloy of tin, silver and gold, which does not deteriorate or discolour in the mouth. It is strong and takes a fine polish, and reproduces the most delicate rugae of the models, thus producing a comfortable and an accurately fitting case. The extra weight of these dentures causes no discomfort after the first few hours.

Difficulties are sometimes met with, especially in cases where a full upper and lower set are worn, in retaining the plates in position during mastication, when a disagreeable noise is occasioned by the teeth striking each other in the act of eating. The addition of a pair of spiral springs to the denture will generally remedy these defects and add materially to the comfort of the patient. Care must of course be taken that the springs do not project and chafe the mucous membrane of the cheeks. Springs are not often required, but where a suction case cannot be successfully worn they form a valuable means of retaining the artificial teeth in position.

Crown and Bridge Work.

"American Dentistry" (?)

ARTIFICIAL teeth may be adapted to the mouth on the suction principle by a closely fitting, skilfully adapted plate, to which the wearer in a few hours becomes perfectly accustomed, or on the crown and bridge principles, by which the artificial teeth are attached to the roots that remain in the mouth.

Crown work is the process of attaching arti-

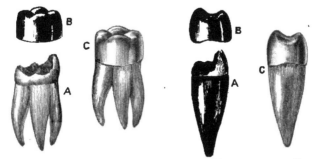

Fig. 76.—A A, Decayed teeth; B B, gold caps; C C, decayed teeth with the gold caps fixed.

ficial crowns to badly decayed teeth, or to roots. There are a number of kinds of crowns used. Those intended for teeth in the anterior part of

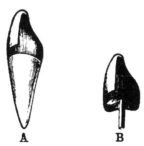

A   B

Fig. 77.—A, Single front tooth crowned; B, artificial crown before fixing on the root.

the mouth are of porcelain, or have porcelain facings, while those employed for back teeth alone are commonly made of gold only.

L

The latter class are caps of gold, which completely envelop and enclose the crown of the tooth, and they are used in those cases in which decay has so wrecked the tooth that a filling would fail to preserve it in a satisfactory condition.

Surrounded by its gold cap the tooth cannot come into contact with foreign substances, so that it is almost impossible for decay to recur.

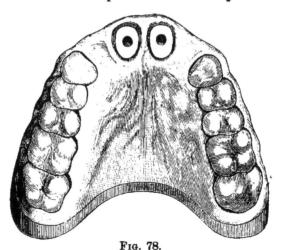

Fig. 78.

Fig. 78 shows a case where four front teeth are missing and the stumps of the central teeth remaining.

For front teeth, crowns with porcelain facings are employed to prevent the unsightly appearance of such an apparent mass of metal. The porcelain facing gives to the tooth a natural appearance. Formerly the work of crowning, which demands great skill and discrimination, was confined mainly to the back teeth; but the modern dentist, having improved methods of manipulation, successfully operates on any tooth if it have but roots which are firmly embedded in the jaw.

BRIDGE WORK.—When there are two or more

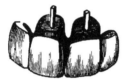

Fig. 79.

Fig. 79 illustrates four artificial teeth constructed for the above mouth on the crown and bridge principle, the plate being entirely dispensed with.

sound roots or teeth, with space from which teeth have been lost between them, it is possible to supply the missing teeth by constructing a

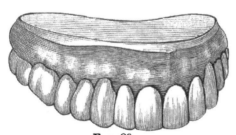

Fig. 80.

Fig. 80 shows the appearance of the same mouth with the denture in position, the four lost teeth being perfectly restored.

bridge of crowns across the vacancy. The crowns are soldered to each other, the terminal ones being firmly attached to the sound teeth or roots in such manner that each of the intermediate crowns occupies the space of a missing

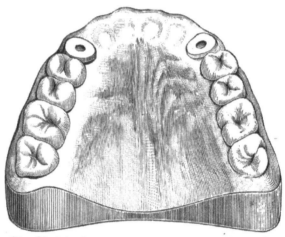

Fig. 81.—Model of case when six front teeth are lost. The stumps of the canines remain.

tooth. They may be constructed with a porcelain facing, so that the whole work shall present to the observer a most natural appearance.

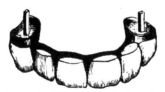

Fig. 82.—Six front teeth prepared for the above case to be attached to canine roots

There are a variety of methods for constructing these bridges, each excellent in itself, and each

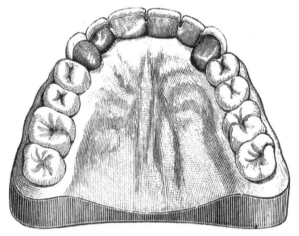

Fɪɢ. 83.—The same case placed in the mouth; there being no plate the palate is uncovered.

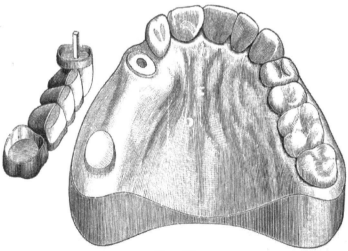

Fɪɢ. 84.

Fig. 84 illustrates a case where four side teeth are lost and a denture constructed to fit attached by a crown covering the last molar, and a cap fitting the root of the canine or eye tooth.

specially adapted to some particular class of cases.

In ordinary bridge work the denture is immovably fixed to the roots or teeth that remain, but artificial cases can be constructed of great strength and durability, easily removable from

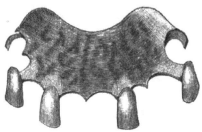

Fig. 85.—Showing a gold case made in the ordinary method.

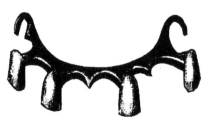

Fig. 86.—Gold case for the same mouth, made as a removable bridge case.

the mouth for purposes of cleaning, etc., and yet possessing the advantages of bridge work as far as the absence of plate is concerned.

Illustrations of these removable bridge or skeleton cases, and of ordinary suction cases constructed for the same mouth show at once the difference between the two methods of fixing artificial teeth.

Bridge work has been condemned by many dentists of high standing because it has been so much abused through its improper use. Some practitioners, from a mistaken enthusiasm have

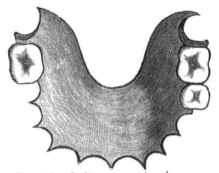

Fig. 87.—Ordinary suction case.

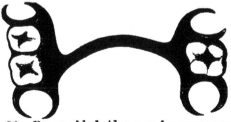

Fig. 88.—Removable bridge case for same mouth.

inserted bridges upon insecure or diseased roots, with the natural consequence of their early failure. Others have not hesitated to sacrifice good and serviceable teeth for the purpose of putting in bridges. All these possible abuses do not excuse the wholesale denunciations of that which is proper and correct practice. As well might one condemn the filling of teeth because poor work is sometimes done. One of the most attractive features of this kind of work is, that when properly made and inserted the patient

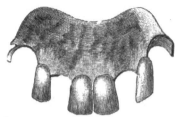

Fig. 89.—Ordinary gold denture.

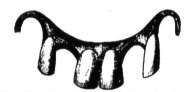

Fig. 90.—Removable bridge denture.

soon loses all consciousness of its artificiality. The crowns and teeth, being attached to natural roots and immovable, approach more nearly to the natural organs, and the patient suffers less discomfort than from any other artificial substitutes. Crown and bridge work has been extensively advertised as American dentistry, but every dentist knows there is nothing in American dentistry to render it different from that

practised in any other country, and that to
speak of American dentistry is as absurd as to
talk of American medicine or surgery, or
American astronomy or any other science.
Modern dentistry, like every art based on
science, owes its perfection to the work of men
of every nationality.   No real man of science,
and no respectable practitioner of any nationality keeps his knowledge secret—to profess to
do so marks a man as a pretender or quack.
Dental science and art cannot be more properly
called American than German, French or
English.

INDEX

Messrs. MATLAND,

Dental Surgeons,

ATTEND AT

1, 3 & 5, FINSBURY PAVEMENT, E.C.

(CORNER of LONDON WALL and FINSBURY PAVEMENT),

From 10 a.m. until 6 p.m.   On Saturdays from
10 a.m. until 2 p.m.

CONSULTATION FREE.